DON'T GET POISONED

D0834833

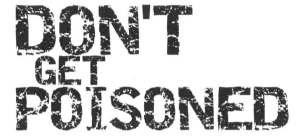

DON'T GET POISONED

PROTECT YOURSELF FROM WILDERNESS TOXINS

Buck Tilton

THE MOUNTAINEERS BOOKS

THE MOUNTAINEERS BOOKS
is the nonprofit publishing arm of The Mountaineers Club, an
organization founded in 1906 and dedicated to the exploration,
preservation, and enjoyment of outdoor and wilderness areas.

1001 SW Klickitat Way, Suite 201, Seattle, WA 98134

© 2010 by Buck Tilton

All rights reserved

First edition, 2010

No part of this book may be reproduced in any form, or
by any electronic, mechanical, or other means, without
permission in writing from the publisher.

Distributed in the United Kingdom by Cordee,
www.cordee.co.uk

Manufactured in the United States of America

Copy Editor: Heath Lynn Silberfeld / enough said
Cover and Book Design: Laura Lind Design
Layout: Laura Lind Design
Cover photographs: © Shutterstock
Illustrations: Moore Creative Design

A catalog record of this book is on file at the Library of
Congress

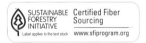

ISBN (paperback): 978-1-59485-339-5
ISBN (e-book): 978-1-59485-412-5

CONTENTS

A NOTE ABOUT SAFETY

Safety is an important concern in all outdoor activities. No book can alert you to every hazard or anticipate the limitations of every reader. The descriptions of techniques and procedures in this book are intended to provide general information. This is not a complete text on any technique. Nothing substitutes for formal instruction, routine practice, and plenty of experience. When you follow any of the procedures described here, you assume responsibility for your own safety. Use this book as a general guide to further information. Under normal conditions, excursions into the outdoors require attention to traffic, road and trail conditions, weather, terrain, the capabilities of your party, and other factors. Keeping informed on current conditions and exercising common sense are the keys to a safe, enjoyable outing.

—*The Mountaineers Books*

INTRODUCTION

The goal of this little book is to provide the knowledge that will make your wilderness trips as totally safe from dangerous poisonings as possible.

One wonders, from time to time, what within the human spirit it is that necessitates a wilderness experience. Leaving behind four walls and a thermostat, we set foot to trail or hand to paddle under skies of blue or gray, or some combination, to be caressed by wind or washed by rain—or blistered by sun or frozen by cold—and it is fun and it is good. We remove out there, somewhere, the taint of polluted air and the cancer of polluted minds. We come home physically tired but mentally and emotionally refreshed, rejuvenated, revitalized. We always come home dirtier on the outside but cleaner on the inside.

At least we *almost* always come home cleaner on the inside.

WHAT IS POISON?

Paracelsus, who died in 1541, was a Swiss physician and botanist who led the way in the use of chemicals in medicine. His pioneering efforts earned him the title "Father of Toxicology." In his words, "Everything is poison, there is poison in everything. Only the dose makes a thing not a poison." Ah, the dose! If *enough* of any substance you ingest, inhale, absorb through your skin, or get injected into your body causes a malfunction in normal biological processes, that substance is called *poison*.

Some poisons rank as highly toxic as even in small amounts they cause a malfunction or two. Others, on the opposite end of the poison spectrum, require quite a high dose to cause a serious threat. But it's not only the dose and potency that make a poison dangerous. Harm to you is also related to your size, age, and general health. In the United States, the greatest number of deaths from poison occurs to small children who swallow something "bad" at home—most often cosmetics, personal care products, and house cleaning products. Fatal inhalations are most likely to involve carbon monoxide, and deadly absorbed poisonings seldom occur outside of industrial or farming settings where strong, toxic chemicals are used. Life-threatening injected poisons are most commonly related to illegal drugs.

When a serious poisoning occurs in the wilderness, it is usually the result of ingesting a poisonous plant, cooking in a tent or snow cave where carbon monoxide builds up, or receiving the bite or sting of a venomous creature.

What to Do: About Poisoning

In general, if you or someone else may have been poisoned, by any route, the first thing you want is information. Through observation or questioning, identify any changes in normal biological processes, which are likely to be characterized by nausea, vomiting, abdominal cramps, diarrhea, muscle cramps, loss of visual acuity, or anything else unusual. Especially indicative of serious poisonings are changes in the level of consciousness (how the brain is working), changes in the respiratory drive (how the lungs are working), or changes in both.

A CLOSER LOOK: Terminology

Toxin usually refers to a potentially dangerous substance found in nature (such as bacteria that cause disease), and *venom* means a specific toxin injected by a bite or sting. But the words *toxic* and *poisonous* are used interchangeably and often; therefore, so are the words *toxin* and *poison*. Don't worry about the meaning. The bottom line is that you don't want problems with poisons, toxins, or venoms.

Shock at a Glance

Many serious poisonings will eventually cause shock. Watch for the following:

- Increasing anxiety, restlessness, or listlessness
- Increasing and weakening heart rate
- Faster and shallower breathing
- Increasingly pale, cool, and sweaty skin

The first-aid measures you can take are covered throughout this book for specific poisons, but all poisoned people should be attended to by a physician. The more pronounced the serious signs and symptoms of poisoning, the more quickly you will want the attention of a medical professional. A doctor (and the poison control center you contact, if you can) will need, or at least greatly desire, the answers to the following questions:

1. What was ingested, inhaled, absorbed, or injected?
2. How much?
3. When?
4. By or into whom (age, body size, overall health)?
5. Why (if known)?

>> IMPORTANT FACT!

You can dial 1-800-222-1222 for the American Association of Poison Control Centers for free, professional advice—24 hours/day, 7 days/week, 365 days/year.

In the wilderness, in fact, fatal poisonings are highly unusual. But since they do happen, you need to be warned, you need to prevent poisonings whenever possible, and you need to know what to do in case of a poisoning. That is what this book is all about.

FASCINATING FACTS

In 2007, the American Association of Poison Control Centers reported more than 4.2 million calls. About 1.6 million calls were requests for information. Approximately 2.5 million calls resulted from a human's exposure to a poison, and 1597 of those humans died.

A CLOSER LOOK: The Numbers
The numbers in this book that relate to data are unreliable in terms of absolute accuracy. Not all poisonings are reportable, and they are, therefore, not all reported. Regional statistics vary. The bottom lines shift season after season, year after year. But the numbers do give an indication of what is happening.

1. INGESTED POISONS

IMAGINE THIS:

Your child wanders into camp chewing and holding half of a little brown mushroom. Your reaction is predictable. Panic! Hours later, still flushed and sweaty and crumpled after a run to the car while carrying the child, a 90-minute drive to the hospital, and a dash into the emergency room, you are trying to make a photo ID of the little brown mushroom from a mycology reference book while the medical staff stands in a corner with heads together, trying to figure out what to do. In the meantime the kid discovers the TV in the waiting room and sits as happy as a pig in truffles. Was your action appropriate?

Swallowing is the most common way for a human to get poisoned. Ingestion, year after year, accounts for approximately 75 to 80 percent of all exposures to poisons. For adults in the United States, the most common ingested poison exposure comes from an overdose of a drug, either prescription or nonprescription, with medications for pain leading the list of human killers. Most of the deaths are accidental.

With ingested poisons, a doctor may ask for specifics: *When did the patient last eat? What else is in the stomach?* And if more than one person in a group suffers: *What possible poison do they have in common?*

FASCINATING FACT

About 10 percent of all poisonings reported to poison control centers in the United States are plant poisonings.

In the outdoors, wild plant ingestions dominate the list of deadly overdoses. What's the risk? In a recent eighteen-year period, thirty documented deaths occurred in people who ate a poisonous plant, with seven of the fatalities blamed on water hemlock, five on jimsonweed, and the rest on a wide variety of potentially dangerous leaves, flowers, roots, berries, and fungi. A vastly larger but unknown number of people, however, got sick. The number of people who consumed a poisonous plant on a wilderness adventure, rather than one from their own backyard, is also unknown but is likely to be extremely small. The reason for this is that most outdoor types follow the Golden Rule of Ingestion: **Eat no wild plant you cannot absolutely identify as safe!**

Not all ingested poisons in the wilderness are plant poisons. Participants on personal and guided outdoor trips may intentionally or unintentionally ingest harmful levels of medications from their own or the group's first-aid kit. Acetaminophen, for example, can be toxic to the liver when taken in large doses. Ibuprofen can be destructive of the kidneys when taken in large doses over a long period of time, and all anti-inflammatory drugs (not just ibuprofen) can cause serious stomach irritation. You need to know the risks involved with drugs you pack, and you need to make sure everyone with access to first-aid kits understands the risks as well.

WATER HEMLOCK

Water hemlock (genus *Cicuta*), considered by many experts to be the most violently poisonous plant in the northern temperate regions of Earth, grows predominantly along waterways and in wet meadows. Hemlocks are tall perennial herbs, members of the carrot family. From the flat-topped clusters of small white flowers, down past the compound leaves with narrow, toothed, pointed leaflets, to the roots that exude a gummy yellow juice when cut, the entire plant is dangerous if ingested. One mouthful of root has been known to kill a large adult. Cicutoxin, the poison in hemlocks, attacks the central nervous system. The one who has

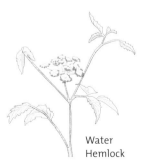

Water
Hemlock

done the ingesting experiences tremors, spasms, convulsions, paralysis, and—if she or he is having a bad day—death. Along the pathway to death, extreme stomach pain, diarrhea, and vomiting are common.

JIMSONWEED

Jimsonweed (*Datura stramonium*) is a plant that grows all over North America and is sometimes known in differing locales as stinkweed, thorn apple, Indian apple, angel's trumpet, sacred datura, and other interesting names. An annual herb, it can grow into a bush that may reach 7 feet in height. Leaves are soft and toothed, and trumpet-shaped flowers bloom in shades of red, pink, yellow, or, by far most familiar, white. Jimsonweed releases a nutlike aroma, especially when crushed. Some people find the smell unpleasant.

Native cultures of the New World used *Datura* to treat venomous snakebites, insect and spider bites, asthma, sore throat, nasal congestion, and bruises. Most often it has been, and still is, used to produce a state of euphoria. It is intentional ingestions, often as a tea made by seekers of a hallucination, that produce most twenty-

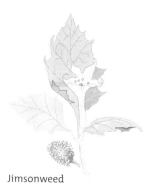

Jimsonweed

first-century jimsonweed poisonings. The leaves and seeds—and to a lesser extent, the roots, stems, and fruit—contain a combination of alkaloids including atropine and scopolamine. These alkaloids are anticholinergics, affecting the nervous system, and in proper doses are often used successfully for medical purposes. In large, uncontrolled doses the chemicals produce delirium, fast heart rates, dilated pupils, and fever. In even larger doses, anticholinergics can produce coma, seizure, respiratory failure, and death.

A CLOSER LOOK: Subtle Seeds

Seeds of apples, apricots, cherries, peaches, and plums contain amygdalin, a cyanogenic glucoside that breaks down in the human digestive tract to release a cyanide. Although the cyanide is of low toxicity, a few fatal encounters have been documented when a large number of seeds were consumed by an individual.

BERRIES

Some berries pack a fatal wallop. Two from deadly nightshade (*Atropa belladonna*), for instance, could kill a child, and ten an adult. Avoid berries that are white, yellow, or green. A few are safe but most are not. About half of all red berries are dangerous to eat, so be sure you can positively identify a red berry before dining. Aggregate berries (each berry looks like a bunch of tiny berries), such as blackberries and thimbleberries, are rarely unsafe to eat. Almost all blue, black, and purple berries—but not entirely all—are safe to eat.

MUSHROOMS

With more than forty thousand known species of fungi on Earth, mushrooms are encountered virtually everywhere people commonly, and sometimes uncommonly, travel. Only a few species are poisonous, and deaths from ingestion are rare, the average running around one fatality per year in the United States. The dead are typically adults and the reason is a case of mistaken identity: gathering the wrong species for dinner or in hopes of a hallucinogenic high.

The mushroom most likely to kill? The *Amanita* (Death Cap, Death Angel, Destroying Angel). Most often growing under deciduous trees in the United States, the several deadly *Amanita* species share characteristics. They show a heavy and typically red, occasionally yellowish to white, and sometimes greenish, cap that can reach 6 inches in width. Thick stalks extend up for 2 to 7 inches with a large bulb at the base. The gills under the cap are usually easily visible and white to green in color. These mushrooms resemble their nickname: toadstool.

The likelihood of post-mushroom ingestion death is about 30 percent in adults and 50 percent in children, and *Amanitas* are responsible for 90 to 95 percent of those deaths. These fungi contain cyclopeptide amatoxins that can produce fatal liver and kidney failure in two to three days. Onset of gastrointestinal distress (severe nausea, vomiting, abdominal cramps, diarrhea) with *Amanita,* and with all potentially death-causing mushrooms, usually falls in the six- to twelve-hour range. After *Amanita* ingestion, in fact, you typically feel fine for at

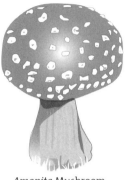

Amanita Mushroom

least four hours, and you may feel fine for up to sixteen hours. After partaking of a mushroom, as a general rule, symptoms that develop within about two hours are unlikely to be from a deadly species. In other words, if stomach discomfort soon follows mushroom munching, the chance of serious mushroom poisoning is extremely slim.

Thus, by the time signs and symptoms show up in serious mushroom poisonings, it's too late to do anything except hurry to a hospital where supportive care might save the life of the consumer. That means if you think someone has eaten a bad 'shroom, *or ingested anything poisonous,* do something to help quickly. If you're in doubt, do something to help quickly. You don't want to wait for a person to look poisoned. With each moment that passes, more and more poison is absorbed.

Note this: If you cannot identify a plant (or any substance) ingested by someone, bring a sample of it to the hospital.

>> *WARNING!*

Although most fatal mushroom encounters involve adults, approximately three out of four mushroom exposures reported to poison control centers occur with children under six years of age. Unlike many products that can poison, wild plants do not come with childproof caps. Adults who take small children into wild areas need to be most aware.

RED TIDE

Sea currents occasionally stir up seeds of dinoflagellates from their repose on the sea floor. These micro-algae may be exposed to enough sunlight and warm surface temperatures to bloom. They live through a single reproductive cycle and drop new seeds to the bed of the ocean where they wait for the next movement of the ever-restless sea. Inside the cell of a limited number of dinoflagellates (such as *Alexandrium catenella*), toxins are produced. The most common toxin encountered in dinoflagellates in the United States is odorless, colorless, and tasteless saxitoxin. If the concentration of these dinoflagellates is high enough, they color the ocean, and you see "red tide." But a red tide does not have to occur for the dinoflagellates to be present in toxic numbers. Many shellfish (oysters, clams, mussels, scallops) store the toxins in their gills and digestive organs while suffering no ill effect. If you eat the toxic shellfish, though, raw or cooked, the result could be paralytic shellfish poisoning.

Shortly after ingestion, tingling starts in the lips and mouth, followed by abdominal cramping, nausea, vomiting, diarrhea, lightheadedness, headache, difficulty with vision, incoherence, and loss of coordination due to a creeping paralysis. The paralysis can affect the ability to breathe enough to cause death. As soon as the signs and symptoms begin to manifest, drink water, swallow some activated charcoal, and head for a hospital.

What to Do: About Ingested Poisons

For someone who has ingested a poison and is still conscious, *limiting the absorption of the poison from the gastrointestinal tract is the prime goal of field management.* Three practical first-aid measures for this situation are available to us in the wilderness: (1) inducing vomiting (with some exceptions), (2) hydrating to dilute the poison, and (3) binding the toxin with activated charcoal.

Dilution is the solution to pollution: Water down, vomit up, or do both for most ingested poisons.

Vomiting

If vomiting can be induced early—the sooner, the better— it may be very beneficial, especially if the ingestion occurred an hour or less prior to treatment. Do the following to induce vomiting:

- Have the person drink a glass, cup, or mug of water.
- Have the person sit up, lean forward, open the mouth, and stick out the tongue.
- Reach in and gently stimulate the gag reflex at the back of the person's throat.
- Stand back.

Don't forget to place the person on his or her left side after vomiting. This puts the end of the stomach, where contents leave for the small intestine, up. In this position gravity works to delay the poison from getting absorbed from the small intestine for up to two hours.

>> *WARNING!*

Syrup of ipecac, a common vomiting inducer, should *not* be used with ingested poisons in the wilderness. It is highly ineffective, and it puts the person at risk if he or she loses consciousness, is unable to protect the airway, and then vomits.

DO *NOT* INDUCE VOMITING IF:
- The person is losing consciousness.
- The person has a seizure disorder or heart problems.
- The person has swallowed corrosive chemicals that can increase damage as they come up.
- The person has swallowed petroleum products that can cause serious pneumonia if even a small amount is breathed into the lungs.

A CLOSER LOOK: Corrosives and Petroleum Products

Corrosive chemicals *are rarely seen* in the wilderness. However, in the occasional case of ingestion of corrosive chemicals, do *not* induce vomiting. Get the person to drink a liter of water or milk (reconstituted powdered milk will work as well as fresh milk). Diluting the poison will reduce its effects.

Petroleum products *are seen* in the wilderness. If someone takes an accidental swallow of white gas, the petroleum product you brought along for your stove, do *not* induce vomiting. White gas ingestion can typically be managed with dilution by drinking a liter of water and without any harm to the patient.

Activated Charcoal

Activated charcoal is postcombustion carbon residue treated to increase its ability to a*d*sorb (not a*b*sorb). In the gastrointestinal tract, poison that has not yet been absorbed by the body will adsorb, or stick to, activated charcoal. When the person next experiences a bowel movement, the poison stuck to the charcoal will pass harmlessly. If swallowed soon after ingestion, activated charcoal may adsorb up to 60 percent of an ingested poison.

With most poisons, even if your care will be short term, binding ingested poisons with activated charcoal is a better treatment than inducing vomiting. By the time you realize you have a poisoned victim, much of the toxin already may have passed out of the stomach. In addition, there are no contraindications for the use of activated charcoal as there are for inducing vomiting. Charcoal may also be administered post-vomiting.

The usual dose of activated charcoal is 50 to 100 grams for adults and 20 to 50 grams for children—but the label on the product you purchase at your local pharmacy will explain further. Although the product is odorless and tasteless, swallowing the slurry of fine black powder may prove to be a chore. The powder can be added to flavored drinks (e.g., fruit drinks), but it should not be mixed with milk or milk products. Charcoal tablets are available for first-aid kits, but they are not recommended for poisonings: the dose is too small to help.

>> CRITICAL POINT!

If someone is found unconscious or goes unconscious, a speedy evacuation to a medical facility is almost always the only life-saving measure to take. Keep unconscious people positioned on their side during the evacuation to maintain their airway.

2. INHALED POISONS

IMAGINE THIS:

Unseasonable snow has kept you and your partner huddled in the tent for almost twenty-four hours. Hunger and thirst have led to firing up the stove under the vestibule, but a fierce wind has driven you and the flaming one-burner inside the tent. Several cups of tea and a freeze-dried dinner later, your mild headache has reached throbbing proportions, and you are thinking your culinary efforts might resurface on the tent floor. Your partner, complaining of head pain earlier, now seems irritable and increasingly confused. What should you do?

When the averages are figured every year, inhalation ends up having caused about 10 percent of all poison exposures. Unlike ingested poisons, inhaled poisons, at least most of them, cause signs and symptoms that appear quickly after exposure. The signs and symptoms show up right away because the poisons (ammonia and chlorine gas are common examples) irritate the eyes, airway, and lungs. In general, watch for burning or watery eyes, coughing, hoarseness, sore throat, and difficult or noisy breathing. Later, maybe, you could observe seizures or altered mental status. The quicker the signs and symptoms show up, the quicker you need to act.

Dilution is the solution to pollution: Get to fresh air fast.

CARBON MONOXIDE

The incomplete combustion of any organic fuel (such as gasoline, kerosene, natural gas, charcoal, wood) results in production of carbon monoxide (CO) gas. Carbon monoxide is invisible, odorless, and tasteless, and once inhaled it enters the bloodstream of the victim where it is approximately 200 times more bondable to the hemoglobin of red blood cells than oxygen. Hemoglobin normally carries oxygen out to the cells of the body. With CO attached, hemoglobin can't carry as much oxygen and can't release what is attached as efficiently. The brain and heart, the organs most in need of a constant flow of oxygen, begin to deteriorate. Tissue death can occur rapidly, and that leads to death of the organism (say, you or your tent partner).

CO is a subtle killer because it does *not* irritate the airway and lungs, and it accounts for approximately one-half the poison deaths in the United States every year. It is the overall leader in death by a specific poison. Most deaths occur in residences and motor vehicles, but CO creates one of the few serious inhaled poison threats on wilderness ventures, especially if you use fuel-burning stoves or lanterns.

FASCINATING FACT
In a recent five-year period, thirty human deaths (and one dog death) were attributed to CO inhalation in tents and campers.

As the amount of attached CO increases in the body to approximately 20 percent of the maximum potential, that person develops a terrible headache, nausea, vomiting, and loss of manual dexterity. At 30 percent, the level of consciousness descends into irritability, impaired judgment, and confusion. It becomes increasingly difficult for the individual to get a full breath, and he or she will grow drowsy. At 40 to 60 percent, the person lapses into a coma. Levels above 60 percent are usually fatal. Death typically results from heart failure. Death by CO is not the pleasant drift into slumber depicted in some movies.

In the field the treatment is simple: move to fresh air! If you have been exposed to low concentrations of CO, you'll probably recover completely in a few hours. The half-life of carbon monoxide attached to hemoglobin runs around five hours. If the concentrations have been high, therefore, you may die even if you are removed from the source of the gas. With high concentrations of CO in the blood, the sufferer needs supplemental oxygen as soon as possible. Breathing 100 percent oxygen—instead of the usual 21 percent available in normal air—reduces the half-life of attached CO to about 60 minutes. Rapid evacuation to a high-pressure chamber, however, may be all that can save a seriously poisoned person. Unconscious victims of CO poisoning will need to have their airway maintained during the evacuation, most easily accomplished by keeping the person in a stable side position.

> ### A CLOSER LOOK: The Gamow Bag
> High-altitude climbers, often tempted to cook in a tent or snow cave, may have a portable high-pressure chamber, the Gamow Bag, available. Unfortunately, it does not create enough pressure to make much of a difference. A high flow of supplemental oxygen is much better.

To avoid hazardous CO exposures, fuel-burning equipment such as camping stoves, camping heaters, lanterns, and charcoal grills should never be used inside a tent, camper, snow cave, or other enclosed shelter. Opening tent flaps, doors, or windows is almost always insufficient to prevent buildup of CO concentrations from these devices. Also, when using fuel-burning devices outdoors, the exhaust should not vent into enclosed shelters.

SMOKE

Annually, deaths due to urban fires are caused—50 to 80 percent of the time—by smoke inhalation and not burns. Serious smoke inhalation in the wilderness, although possible, is rare. Smoke is a mixture of heated particles and gases, and the threat, impossible to determine for sure, is directly related to what is being burned, how hot it is burning, and how much oxygen is available to feed the burning. As with other dangerous inhalations, watch for coughing, shortness of breath, hoarseness, headache, and changes in mental status. If persistent, these signs and symptoms require an evacuation of the inhaler.

DESERT FUNGUS

Two fungi found from time to time in desert soil (soil that is dry, gets little rainfall, sits low in elevation, and experiences high summer temperatures)—including soil in parts of America's Southwest—can cause illness and possibly death. They are the only two species of the genus *Coccidioides,* the spores of which, if inhaled, cause a disease known as coccidioidomycosis. The spores get airborne when kicked up by winds or aggressive movement of the soil by humans, such as agricultural pursuits or possibly a group of hikers trampling heavily. In most people the spores cause an upper respiratory infection, usually described as something on the low end of severe, but it then resolves harmlessly, leaving the patient immune to future contact. However, if an abundant number of spores are inhaled—which they rarely are—a fatal form of the disease can occur, in which the spores migrate to the brain and other important places. If you get really sick, find a doctor.

What to Do: About Inhaled Poisons

Whether breathed in accidentally or intentionally (almost always for some sort of "high"), inhaled poisons enter the blood where they do their nasty deeds and where they cannot be removed. All you can do is immediately remove the person from the source of the poison, prevent any further exposure to the poison, make sure fresh air surrounds the person, and find a source of high-concentration/high-flow supplemental oxygen as soon as possible. Seriously threatened people, in other words, need a quick trip to the nearest hospital. And if they stop breathing on the way there, they will need rescue breathing.

A CLOSER LOOK: Inhaled Insect Repellents

Some insect repellents are highly toxic if inhaled, and those containing DEET and permethrin are the most notable. Those expelled in aerosol form or from pump sprays are the risky ones. Safety lies in products that you smear on from containers or wipe on with pads or cloths. Fresh air is the only available treatment in the wild.

3. ABSORBED POISONS

IMAGINE THIS:

After a long afternoon on a summer trail, you drop your pack and plop down in the shade of tall trees. A stream gurgles along happily near your feet, the air further cooled by the closeness of the water. You are fingering the green foliage sprouting luxuriantly close to the ground all around when suddenly it dawns on you: leaves of three! What should you do?

Many substances can enter your body by being absorbed through your skin. Those substances that are "poisonous" fall, generally speaking, into two categories: (1) those that cause mild to extensive local damage and (2) those that work their way harmfully into your critical biological functions. The poisons that cause local damage, from irritations to serious burns, include strong acids, alkalis, and some hydrocarbons—and they can be extremely damaging. Pesticides and some industrial chemicals sit at the top of the dangerous list of those that can kill you, some rather quickly.

A rash, itching and burning skin, swelling, and blisters could indicate contact with an absorbed poison. Fever, headache, and overall weakness are possible when the poison causes systemic malfunctions. Later you might have difficulty breathing and an increased heart rate. Once again, the faster the signs and symptoms appear, the faster you need to act.

The basics of how to act with absorbed poisons include the following:

1. Remove contaminated clothing and all clothing that could be contaminated, but take steps to prevent further contamination. Wear gloves.
2. Use absorbent material immediately to soak up liquid poisons. Wear gloves.
3. Brush off dry poisons. Wear gloves.
4. Flush skin with fresh water for ten minutes. For strong alkalis, do a twenty-minute flush. If you're unsure, flush for twenty minutes.
5. After thorough flushing, wash with soap and water.
6. Get the poisoned person to a doctor.

>> WARNING!

Some dangerous substances, such as phosphorous and elemental sodium, react violently when they get wet. They burn skin. These substances can only be—and should be—brushed off.

POISON IVY, POISON OAK, AND POISON SUMAC

The greatest risk by far of an absorbed poison in the wild arises from poisonous plants that cause a reaction usually limited to skin level. The offending plants are most often poison ivy, poison oak, or poison sumac, and all three are members of the genus

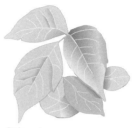

Poison Ivy

Toxicodendron. These poisonous plants grow all over the United States except in Alaska and Hawaii, but you rarely find them above approximately 5000 feet elevation, in deserts, or in rainforests. Near water, especially if it's hot and sunny, they'll grow abundantly. Generally speaking, in the United States poison ivy grows east of the Rocky Mountains, poison oak west of the Rockies, and poison sumac in the southeastern states.

So, what do they look like? Appearances vary, and identification can be a problem for the untrained. Poison ivy can look like a small shrub as well as a woody, ivylike vine; poison oak typically is a shrub; poison sumac is a shrub or tree that prefers

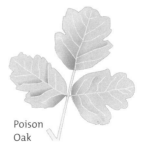

Poison Oak

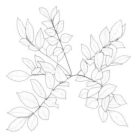

Poison Sumac

marshy ground and reaches as high as 40 feet but averages around 15 feet. The leaves of any of these may be smooth edged, sawtooth edged, or lobed, and the leaves may be rough, smooth, or hairy. Poison ivy and oak leaves do indeed *almost* always grow in threes with the middle leaf extending farther than the other two. Poison sumac grows in a complex leaf of seven to thirteen paired and pointed leaflets. The message here is that you must learn to identify the members of this genus that grow in your area because what all *Toxicodendron* species share in common, without any exceptions, is urushiol.

A CLOSER LOOK: Toxicodendron Identification
As an adjunct to classic methods of plant identification, you can use this test to identify members of the genus *Toxicodendron*. Several leaves from the offending plant can be crushed on a piece of white paper—carefully, so as not to contaminate your fingers or clothes! (Wear rubber gloves or plastic bags on your hands.) If the sap stain markedly darkens within a few minutes, the plant is very likely poisonous.

Urushiol and the Reaction

Not only the leaves but practically the entire *Toxicodendron* plant contains urushiol, a heavy oil, which is an evil substance that initiates a contact dermatitis, a sequence of skin reactions leading to the foul, oozing bumps that itch sufficiently to drive the most stoic round the bend. Urushiol is usually colorless (sometimes light yellow), and it is potent stuff. In the very sensitive person, just 2-millionths to 2.5-millionths of a gram will trigger a reaction, and about 50 percent of all adults in the United States are very sensitive. Another 35 percent will have a reaction to higher concentrations. The rest do not react, even to extremely high concentrations. No one knows why some people are tolerant of urushiol—perhaps an acquired immunity, perhaps a genetic blessing—but, without a doubt, sensitivity to the oil is the single most common source of allergic skin reactions in the United States and perhaps the whole world.

When urushiol soaks into human skin, it binds at benzene ring positions to surface proteins of certain cells and well, um, to make a long story short, an allergic reaction takes place. Not everyone reacts exactly the same, but most people first develop redness where they contacted the oil. The redness often appears in streaks where the plant brushed the skin. Swelling may occur. Blisters, sometimes large, sometimes small, erupt later and discharge the fluid that fills them. The discharge will eventually form a firm crust. Unless you've spent your entire life north of the Arctic Circle, you already know the entire area itches with indescribable ferocity.

A CLOSER LOOK: Urushiol De-Mythed

Scratching the blisters open does not spread the poison. The fluid in the blisters is harmless, but you can spread the oil easily when it gets on your hands, causing the rash to show up in places you know never touched a plant.

Wind cannot carry urushiol. It's too heavy. But smoke particles can if you burn a plant in a fire. You could even inhale smoke-borne particles and suffer a devastating airway reaction, treatable only in a hospital.

After contact, it takes varying amounts of time for the reaction to show up. On thicker areas of the body, such as hands and feet, the oil soaks in more slowly than on thinner areas. Still, for sensitives, the bad stuff begins to happen in two to six hours. Those with low sensitivity may not develop signs or symptoms for days or as long as two weeks. For most people, twelve to forty-eight hours brings assurance that the next ten days to two weeks or more will be cursed with the misery of the reaction. Adding agony to misery, parts of the body that have reacted in the past could fire up again when a new body part reacts to a fresh contact.

In terms of stability, urushiol finds few equals, being found active in dried plants dating back more than a hundred years. Stomp through, say, a patch of poison oak, and store your boots for a couple of years. Slip back into your boots, and you could suddenly react to poison ivy. You can pick up the oil from your clothing, the bottom of your tent, your hiking staff, or the hair of your dog or cat. Neither dog nor cat, by the way, nor any other critter, seems to react to urushiol—humans only.

Good news: The oil is contained within the plant, not on the surface, which means casually brushing against an intact *Toxicodendron* will not spread urushiol on your skin. Bad news: The plant may not be intact, even though it appears so, for many reasons, such as a previous hiker stomping the plants, a bug chewing the plants, or a strong wind whipping the leaves wildly to and fro.

An allergen for all seasons, urushiol remains equally devastating throughout the year. Beware, therefore, even the brown stems and roots of winter and the red leaves of fall if they're still attached to the stems. Plant juices return to stems and roots in the fall, leaving dead leaves littering the ground with virtually no urushiol in them.

What to Do: Treatment of Absorbed Poisons

Nothing cures an urushiol rash, but you'll assuredly want to try several methods of relieving the itch. Aspirin, nonsteroidal anti-inflammatory drugs (such as ibuprofen), and oral antihistamines have no effect, although the antihistamine might enable you to sleep better. Topical lotions, creams, or sprays that contain antihistamines or anesthetics (words that usually end in *-caine*) should be avoided since the additives have a tendency to make things worse. Topical corticosteroids sold over the counter are too weak to work well. Your physician may be able to prescribe a strong topical steroid that will work, if you start using it before the reaction has turned to blisters. Topical applications of calamine lotion usually reduce the itch. Soaking in a tepid bath with two cups of Linit starch added usually reduces the itch. A cold wet compress sometimes brings relief, but, on the other end of the heat spectrum, many sufferers report substantial aid from standing in a hot shower for several minutes, then gently patting the water off the itchy area. But you don't need a shower. Simply soaking the affected body parts in water as hot as tolerable often provides anti-itch relief for hours, but the hot water soak must follow a thorough cleaning of the affected area of the body to remove the oil (see "What to Do: Prevention of Absorbed Poisons").

FASCINATING FACT
Home remedies abound, with recipes for folk medications against the itch numbering more than a hundred. If you've tried one, and it works for you, keep using it.

Natural Remedies
There are two plants whose juices may ease the torment. Plantain, both the common and buckhorn

variations, has leaves that release a pale green sap when crushed. Dabbed on the rash, plantain sap reportedly stops the itch for twenty-four to forty-eight hours. Common plantain has broad, irregularly rounded or oval-ish leaves,

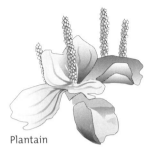

Plantain

1 to 6 inches long, that grow in a rosette near the ground. The leaves of buckhorn plantain are more lance-like in shape. A spike rises as much as 12 inches from the center of the rosette, covered in inconspicuous flowers and then seeds.

The second plant, jewelweed, has as many advocates as plantain. Once again, the juice from crushed plants is applied to the rash with what you pray will be helpful results. Jewelweed supporters also claim satisfaction from soaking in a tub of water to which the juice of approximately one pound of the plant has been added. Jewelweed grows 3 to 5 feet tall with oval-shaped leaves that are round-toothed along the edges. The flowers, sort of trumpet-shaped,

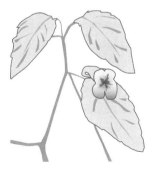

Jewelweed

dangle from the plant a bit like jewels from a necklace and are either pale yellow or orange with red dots, depending on the species. The orange-flowered variety works better for the treatment of Toxicodendron poisoning.

>> *WARNING!*

Forgo self-treatment and hastily find a doctor if you swell significantly; if your airway, face, or genitals are involved; or if any other reaction that seems serious to you erupts.

What to Do: Prevention of Absorbed Poisons

In addition to recognition and avoidance of *Toxicodendron* species, several actions may prevent the reaction after contact is made. Of prime importance is washing as soon as possible after you realize you may have touched one of these poisonous plants. Even the extremely sensitive have an estimated five minutes to wash off the urushiol before it soaks in enough to cause trouble. Cold water, lots and lots of it, inactivates urushiol, so plunging into a nearby stream or lake, depending on your ability to swim, would be a reasonable act. Experts say that if you have plenty of cold water available, especially within the first three minutes of contact, soap does not help. Avoid hot water, which may spread the oil around more than rinse it off during the washing process.

Washing with soap and water after exposure to urushiol goes back to at least the 1930s, and soap is still recommended by many dermatologists after the three-minute period ends. As to what kind of soap, the experts vary in exact recommendations, but detergents—such as dish and laundry—seem to work as well as anything. Wash gently and repeatedly, six or seven times, and rinse thoroughly in between.

Dilution is the solution to pollution: Wash off absorbed poisons.

FASCINATING FACT

Barrier creams, substances applied topically to block or retard absorption of urushiol, are available. They must be applied *before* contact.

Organic solvents such as alcohol and gasoline may wash off urushiol better than water or soap and water. The preferred method is to dab repeatedly with several pieces of solvent-soaked cotton to pick up urushiol from the skin before giving your skin a good rub with fresh solvent-soaked cotton. Once the solvent dries, urushiol caught in the cotton will redeposit on your skin, so don't use the same piece of cotton for more than a few moments. Solvents are especially useful for removing urushiol from gear.

When you wash your hands, be sure to clean under your fingernails.

Remember to wash any clothes that may be contaminated. Clothing may hold the oil, protecting your skin at first, but the oil will remain active for a long, long time, returning to haunt you with the aggravating itch if you don't wash that shirt thoroughly.

>> WARNING!

Despite what you might have heard, you *cannot* eat little bits of poison ivy, oak, or sumac from time to time to slowly develop immunity.

4. INJECTED POISONS

IMAGINE THIS:

Your neck is stiff and other muscles ache. You have a low fever and unusual fatigue. All things considered, you feel crummy—as bad as or worse than you did with some kind of flu last year. But the frightening thing about this illness is the red rash that keeps appearing, growing, and fading—and the rash causes you pain. Should you find a doctor?

Looking at the big poison picture in the United States, serious injected poison exposures—and death—are almost always the result of substance abuse, with heroin and cocaine sitting year after year, almost unbelievably—you'd think people would know better—at the top of the list. In the outdoors, bites and stings create the potential for danger.

Some animals inject venoms: poisons that vary greatly in severity depending on the species of animal, the way the human acts during and after the confrontation, and, sometimes, the reason for the attack. Some animals inject toxins: poisons that may cause diseases.

Every year *millions* of people on Earth die because they were bitten (and if you read on, you'll learn why). In the United States, however, your chance of death by bite or sting is small—some would say extremely small. But your chance of avoiding a bite or sting a time or two, or dozens of times, is virtually nonexistent. Since numerous biters and stingers are out there, and the poisons they carry are numerous, and what you should do varies, this chapter is the longest in this book. Despite its length, it does not address all possible bites and stings—just the most common.

REPTILES

Generally speaking, snakes will put considerable effort into avoiding humans and bite only when threatened. But if they do bite, an estimated 15 percent of about 3000 species of snakes on Earth may be considered potentially dangerous to human beings. Some of the best guesses by experts place the number of deaths each year, worldwide, as high as 125,000. Available data offer unreliable statistics since snakebites are not reportable injuries, but know this for sure: few of these snake-caused deaths occur in the United States. Out of an estimated 7000 to 8000 or so venomous snakebites per year in the United States, there may be, when the snakes have a good year, say some experts, fifteen bites fatal to humans. The number probably stands much lower for most recent years—five to six deaths per year say other experts. The low number of

VENOMOUS SNAKES OF THE WORLD

Family	Subfamily	Examples	Characteristics
Viperidae	Crotalinae	All the pit vipers: Bushmasters Copperheads Cottonmouths Fer-de-lances Rattlesnakes etc.	Heat-sensitive pit between eye and nostril; catlike pupils; retractable fangs
Viperidae	Viperinae	All the true vipers: Gaboon vipers Puff adders Russell's vipers Saw-scaled vipers etc.	No heat-sensitive pit
Elapidae		Cobras Coral snakes Kraits Mambas etc.	Short, fixed fangs; chewing some-times required to inject venom
Hydro-phidae		All true sea snakes: Pelagic sea snake etc.	Fangs similar to snakes in Elapidae family

deaths can be accredited, most likely, to the availability of effective antivenins and the relatively low toxicity of the venom of snakes in the United States.

At least ninety-nine out of every one hundred poison-ous bites by indigenous snakes in the United States are received from a pit viper, family Viperidae: rattlesnakes, copperheads, and water moccasins (also known as cot-tonmouths). The other bite usually comes from a coral snake, family Elapidae, or from poisonous exotic snakes being kept as pets. Almost all the fatalities caused by snakes in the United States occur after a bite from either an eastern or a western diamondback rattlesnake. Those who die are usually very young, very old, or unable to find a source of antivenin.

Facts about the number of lizard bites in the United States are even less reliable than for snakebites. In all the world, however, only two lizards are venomous. Both are found in North America, and both are of the genus *Heloderma*. One, the Gila monster, is relatively common in the United States.

Pit Vipers

Widely dispersed, all rattlesnakes are pit vipers (subfamily Crotalinae), and they are by far the most common of at least thirty-four species of pit vipers in North America —but not all pit vipers have rattles. Copperheads and water moccasins are rattle-less, and newborn rattlesnakes cannot make the distinctive "buzz" until after their first shedding of skin even though they can bite and inject venom prior to growing grown-up rattles. All pit vipers *do* have distinctly triangular heads, catlike pupils, heat-sensitive pits between eyes and nostrils (thus the name "pit viper"), and danger squirting from two very special fangs hinged to swing downward at a 90-degree angle from the upper jaw. At rest the fangs fold against the roof of the snake's mouth. At unrest the jaw opens alarmingly wide and the fangs drop into striking position, allowing

VENOM DELIVERY APPARATUS OF A PIT VIPER

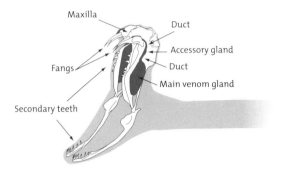

Maxilla

Duct

Accessory gland

Duct

Fangs

Main venom gland

Secondary teeth

the venom to be ejected via muscular contraction down canals within the fangs and into the tissue of prey or an enemy when the snake bites. Both the upright position of the fangs and the injection of venom are controlled by the "will" of the snake: it can open its mouth without showing the fangs, and it can bite without injecting venom. In short, pit vipers have the most sophisticated venom delivery system in the entire snake world.

Somewhere between 75 and 80 percent of pit viper bites are associated with envenomation. Or, to say it another way, one out of every four to five bites is "dry": no venom is injected. Why? Who knows for sure? The snake may have used its venom recently, and it takes time to biologically manufacture more. The snake may instinctively know a human, even dead, will remain inedible, and it may choose to save its venom for mealtime. How upset, startled, or frightened the snake is may also be a factor in (1) whether it injects venom or not and (2) how much venom it injects.

Venom or no venom, all victims have in common one or two things: fang marks. One fang mark means either the snake lost a fang prior to biting or missed with the other fang when it did bite. You may see small marks from the snake's secondary teeth as well.

>> WARNING!

Pit vipers come in all sorts of sizes, colors, and distinctive patterns along their lengths. It is beyond the scope of this little book to attempt to describe them specifically. Check with local experts to learn descriptions of local dangerous snakes in areas where you intend to travel.

Pit Viper Envenomation

Pit viper venom, a very complex poison, acts aggressively on local tissue, "digesting" it, sort of—a fact that makes the normal prey of the snake easier to process as food. Systemic effects—things that happen away from the bite site—in victims are also common.

How dangerous is pit viper venom to a human? The amount of venom and the toxicity of the venom are primary factors determining the risk to the bitten. Poison from the Mojave rattlesnake, for instance, rates as approximately forty-four times more potent than

the Southern copperhead's. Risk factors also include
(1) the size and health of the snake, (2) the age, size,
health, and emotional stability of the victim, (3) where,
anatomically, the bitten got bitten, (4) how deep the
fangs went, (5) the first aid provided, and (6) the hospital
care provided.

A CLOSER LOOK: Pit Viper Danger Zones

Historically, the five states in which you are most
likely to receive a fatal snakebite are these, listed
from most likely to least likely:

1. Arizona   4. Texas
2. Florida   5. Alabama
3. Georgia

The results of envenomation vary greatly, depending
on the variables noted above. No precise way to
differentiate the seriousness of a pit viper bite exists, but
generally speaking, the following statements are true:

• *Mild pit viper envenomations* (about 35 percent of all
envenomations) usually cause severe burning pain
within minutes. You can, however, not hurt much
and still be significantly poisoned, depending mostly
on the species that bit you. Within thirty to sixty
minutes other signs and symptoms may develop.
Variable swelling progresses outward from the bite.
Variable ecchymosis (black and blue bruising) often
appears. Blood may keep oozing from the wound as a

result of the anticoagulant effect of the venom. Common are nausea with or without vomiting, weakness, dizziness or faintness, sweating and chills, and numbness or tingling of the mouth, tongue, scalp, or feet. A strange taste in the mouth, such as "metallic" or "rubbery," may be described.

- *Moderate pit viper envenomations* (about 25 percent of the total) may include all the above, except worse, with the addition of swelling that moves up the arm or leg toward the heart and swollen lymph nodes along the way. Ecchymosis sometimes develops at anatomic locations somewhat remote from the bite.
- *Severe pit viper envenomations* (about 10 to 15 percent of the total) could be indicated by all the above, except even worse, and can add big jumps in pulse rates and breathing rates, profound swelling, blurred vision, headache, and shock.

Another way to evaluate the severity of a pit viper bite is this: the sooner the bad things start happening postbite and the more profound the bad things, the worse the envenomation. Death is possible in severe cases.

>> WARNING!

Many of the symptoms of a snakebite are directly proportional to the fear the victim experiences. If bitten, staying as calm as possible is decidedly in your best interest.

When the Snake Bites. At dawn and dusk, during the warmest months—April to September in the United States—when snakes are most active (and humans, perhaps, more careless), you are most likely to get bitten.

>> *WARNING!*
A dead, even decapitated pit viper can reflexively bite and inject venom for up to one hour after death.

Where and Who the Snake Bites. As you move south geographically into warmer territory, you find increasing numbers of snakes and correspondingly increasing numbers of snake-bitten humans. Bites occur most often to the lower extremities with upper extremities coming in second. Upper extremity bites are usually from a harassed snake: someone has tried to kill it, capture it, or otherwise handle it. The most common profile of a bitten human in the United States is this: a young, intoxicated male, seventeen to twenty-seven years of age, who intentionally messes with a pit viper.

What to Do: Pit Viper Bites

Antivenins are available, often readily available in hospitals near snake country. Most victims of snakebite, in the meantime, will benefit from the following guidelines, which have been developed especially for North American pit viper envenomation. Please notice that there are almost as many *do not's* as there are *do's*. The *do not's* are important because they can make the victim quite a bit worse when undertaken.

1. Calm and reassure the victim.
2. Keep the victim physically at rest with the bitten extremity immobilized and kept at approximately the same level as the heart.
3. Remove rings, watches, and anything else that might reduce local circulation if swelling occurs.
4. Gently wash the wound.
5. Measure the circumference of the extremity at the site of the bite and at a couple of sites between the bite and the heart, and monitor swelling.
6. Evacuate the victim by carrying, or going for help to carry, or, if the victim is stable, by slow walking with frequent rest breaks.
7. If the victim is kept still, keep the victim warm.
8. Keep the victim well hydrated with clear fluids unless he or she develops pronounced vomiting.
9. Do NOT cut or suck (even with a suction device).
10. Do NOT apply ice or immerse the wound in icy water.
11. Do NOT apply a tourniquet.
12. Do NOT give the victim alcohol to drink.
13. Do NOT electrically shock the victim.

A CLOSER LOOK: Crotalid Antivenin

Old antivenins are made from horse serum, and allergic reactions, sometimes severe, are common. The newest antivenin utilizes sheep serum and promises far fewer adverse reactions. In addition, the newest antivenin is more broadly targeted and should also work for cottonmouth and copperhead bites instead of primarily for rattlesnake bites. The recommended dose for treating a victim with the antivenin varies depending on the physician's assessment of the severity. And it's expensive, sometimes costing more than $17,000 for treatment with new antivenin.

North American Pit Vipers: Facts, Not Myths

1. Pit vipers, all species considered, hit maximum crawl speed at about 3 miles per hour (5 kilometers per hour), no faster than an adult's determined walking rate.
2. Pit vipers do not chase humans, although they may get confused and slither *toward* a human.
3. Pit viper fangs grow no longer than 0.8 inch (20 mm) even in the largest rattlesnakes.
4. Pit vipers strike at a maximum speed of about 8 feet per second.
5. Pit vipers can strike distances of no more than approximately one-half their own body length.
6. Pit vipers use their forked tongue only (and harmlessly) to detect chemical odors in the environment.
7. Pit vipers that have rattles do not always use them before they strike.

8. Pit viper babies are, perhaps, more likely to strike, but an adult snake can inject an average of seventeen times more venom than a baby, and that makes the adult far more dangerous.

9. Pit vipers, namely the eastern diamondback rattlesnake, can exceed 6.5 feet (2 meters) in length.

Coral Snakes

The bands of color on coral snakes (subfamily Viperinae) completely encircle the snake's body. Brightly banded in red, yellow, and black, all coral snakes of the United States are described by a particular color sequence: "Red on black, venom lack; red on yellow, kill a fellow." In other words, red bands bordered by yellow bands indicate danger. (Please note that dangerous snakes resembling coral snakes of the United States that are found *outside* the United States do not always obey the above color rule.) Coral snakes are found in Arizona, Texas, and the southeastern states in three subspecies that resemble each other very much.

Since coral snakes cannot strike out as pit vipers do, most coral snake bites are the reward a human receives for handling a coral snake. Even then their short, fixed fangs in the front of a small mouth make it all but impossible for coral snakes to bite anything on humans other than a finger, a toe, or a fold in the skin, and they almost always have to hang on and chew to do damage. You may have ample time, and you are well advised, to snatch off a chewing coral snake before it chews long enough to inject a significant amount of venom. Approximately 40 percent of coral snake bites envenomate the bitten.

Experts disagree over the number of coral snake bites to humans occurring annually, with ranges varying from about twenty to around sixty. Who knows when the last human death from a bite occurred? It could have been over fifty years ago. No confirmed human deaths have occurred since development of the antivenin.

A CLOSER LOOK: You Are Alone
Alone and bitten? Follow all the management guidelines with one exception: you *should* walk out slowly with frequent rest breaks. Do not wait around to see if you are going to swell up or die.

Coral Snake Envenomation
On the complexity scale, coral snake venom ranks much lower than pit viper venom. On the potency scale, however, these colorful reptiles are much higher. In the United States only the Mojave rattler has more potent venom than a coral snake, and one adult coral snake packs enough venom to kill four to five adult humans. Fortunate it is that these snakes are shy, nonaggressive, and poorly adapted to bite humans.

Once bitten the victim may or may not complain of pain, mild and soon going away. Localized swelling is possible but not common. It takes as much as twelve to thirteen hours for signs and symptoms to reach the point where the victim wants help. Then you might hear complaints of nausea followed by vomiting, often the earliest sign and symptom. Headache, stomach pain, and sweaty and pale skin are common. Be alert for dizziness, weakness, numbness, and difficulty speaking and swallowing. Respiratory difficulty and an altered mental status (such as drowsiness) are really bad signs. Despite the fact that deaths are rare, it is estimated that untreated coral snake bites would kill about 10 percent of the bitten.

>> *WARNING!*
From a very safe distance, try to identify any snake that bites, but do not attempt to catch the snake. Of such behavior are second victims created.

What to Do: Coral Snake Bites

Since significant signs and symptoms can be long delayed, early evacuation of persons suspected of having been bitten by coral snakes is strongly advised. How you get a victim to a doctor does not seem to matter much, but speed does. Antivenin should be started as soon as possible to be most effective. Little first aid works other than keeping the patient calm and cleaning the wound—with one possible exception: the pressure-immobilization technique. Developed in Australia

THE PRESSURE-IMMOBILIZATION TECHNIQUE

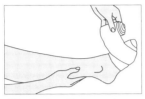

a) Starting from the toes, put a broad, firm bandage around the bitten area. Don't take off any clothes such as jeans, but cut the seams if they can't be pushed out of the way, and keep the leg as still as possible while you are bandaging.

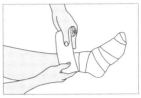

b) Make the bandage as tight as for a sprained ankle.

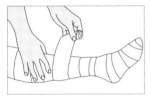

c) Bandage as much of the leg as possible, especially the toes.

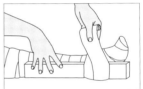

d) Put a splint beside the bandage and bind that to the leg to help keep the leg still.

where numerous relatives of the coral snake live and bite, pressure-immobilization involves securing elastic wraps (such as those used to secure sprained ankles) around the bite site, up the extremity, and back down the extremity, followed with some type of splint. Properly applied—with about the same pressure as wrapping a sprained ankle—pressure-immobilization prevents the spread of Elapid venom until a hospital can be found.

It has proven very effective as first aid for Elapid bites in Australia but remains untested on coral snake bites. It could, however, help a lot.

A CLOSER LOOK: Potency of Snake Venom

Snake venom may be rated according to the amount required to provide a lethal dose (LD) to 1 kilogram (32.15 ounces) of mice. From most dangerous to least dangerous:

Australia's small-scaled (fierce) snake venom LD = 0.01 mg

India's Indian cobra venom LD = 0.50 mg

America's rattlesnake (average) venom LD = 11.40 mg

Gila Monsters

With about 3000 species of lizards known today, it is somewhat surprising, despite plenty of mythology to the contrary, that only the Gila (hee-lah) monster and the Mexican beaded lizard are venomous. Be that as it may, Gila monsters live quiet and peaceful lives, if undisturbed, hunting at night throughout much of the southwestern United States and growing to a maximum length of less than two feet. They are essentially black with smears of yellow, pink, or both. Built like weight lifters of the lizard world, they also have especially massive jaw muscles. Their powerful jaws compensate for primitive teeth and no means to inject their poison. The venom glands of these lizards are in their lower jaws and not connected to their teeth (as in snakes). They lock on when they bite while the venom drools into the wound they create, making removal of the lizard from your hand or foot highly advisable but often difficult to achieve.

Gila monsters would not cause much pain when they bite except that they hang on so tight and chew so hard. They move sluggishly and never bite humans unless they are messed with—by being picked up or stepped on—at which time they are capable of pivoting rapidly in your hand or on their hind legs and lashing out with surprising speed.

Gila Monster Envenomation

Gila monster venom is comparable to coral snake venom, but these lizards produce very little of it. Bleeding from the nasty wound of the bite may be more arresting initially. Pain, throbbing or burning, may radiate up an arm or leg. Envenomation may produce nausea and vomiting, dizziness and weakness, profuse sweating, and difficulty breathing. On the plus side, it has been at least fifty years since a confirmed human death in the United States from a Gila monster bite—and some experts believe even that death might not have been from a Gila monster.

What to Do: Gila Monster Bites

You may likely be required to heat the underside of a Gila monster's jaws with matches or a lighter, place the attached lizard under a flow of hot water, or pry open the jaws with some instrument to break its grip—and doing so should be your first management procedure. Stop the bleeding with direct pressure and, afterward, thoroughly clean the bite wound. Splint the wounded area and find a doctor. Nothing else of importance in terms of care need be noted here.

>> WARNING!

Gila monsters freed from attachment to a victim have immediately turned the rescuer into a second victim.

A CLOSER LOOK: Gila Monsters De-Mythed

1. *They do not have poisonous breath.*

2. *They cannot spit their venom.*

3. *They are not able to sting with their tails.*

4. *They will not hold on when they bite until it thunders—maybe.*

What to Do: Prevention of Reptile Bites

1. Do not try to pick up or otherwise try to capture snakes or lizards.

2. Check places you intend to put your hands and feet before exposing your body part to a potential bite, especially in the dark.

3. Gather firewood before dark, or do it carefully while using a flashlight.

4. In snake country, keep your tent zipped up.

5. Wear high, thick boots and/or gaiters while traveling in dangerous snake and lizard country.

6. When passing a snake, stay out of striking range,
which is about one-half the snake's length.

7. If you hear the "buzz" of a rattler, freeze, find it with
your eyes without moving your head, wait for it to
relax the strike position, and back away slowly.

ARACHNIDS

Being an arachnid means having eight legs (four pairs
of them). It also means being a member of the largest
noninsect class of arthropods (invertebrates with an
exoskeleton). Being an arachnid does not necessarily
mean being a spider. It could, for instance, mean being
a tick or a scorpion, and those two are discussed later
in this chapter.

A few people know, and those who do not are seldom
gladdened to learn, that most spiders, worldwide,
carry venom that can be injected through nasty fangs.
Furthermore, all spiders are carnivorous and spend
their lives waiting for or hunting for living prey.
Their venom is designed to paralyze and liquefy the
tissues of their prey so the spider can then ingest the
tissues. Spider venom dangerous to humans, then,
causes predictable results: pain, the death of local
tissue, or both.

On the positive side, only a few dozen species of
spiders on Earth have a bite harmful to humans. In the

United States, medical significance applies to only three spiders: widows, browns, and hobos. Most spiders are harmless to you because they either (1) have venom that does not work on mammals, (2) have too little venom to bother mammals, or (3) have fangs that cannot penetrate mammalian, including human, skin.

Widow Spiders

The widows (genus *Latrodectus*), at least five species of which are found in North America, are spiders common around the globe. In the United States almost everyone is familiar with the black widow, an inhabitant of every state but Alaska. But one North American species of widow spider is brown, and one species is called the red-legged spider.

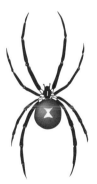

Black Widow Spider (underside view)

Only the females are dangerous to humans. The dark, shiny female black widow, the one most often recognized, may reach 2 inches (4 to 5 cm) in leg span, and she packs a remarkable potency in every little bit of venom. Drop for drop, widow venom is stronger than most rattlesnake venom. Her venom's potential for harm makes her the most dangerous of spiders found in North America. The typically red—but not always red—

"hourglass" shape on the underside of her abdomen helps identify her. In some species, however, the two sides of the "hourglass" fail to meet, so two triangles almost joining are seen. Males, by the way, are smaller (about one-third the size of females) and lighter in color with even lighter markings and a faint "hourglass." Males cannot bite through human skin.

The female widow spider hides her tattered web under logs and large pieces of bark, in stone crevices, in trash heaps and outbuildings, and deep in clumps of heavy vegetation—and she infrequently leaves it. Rarely aggressive, she may be touchy during springtime mating and egg-tending days. Even then, she seldom bites unless she senses a threat to her web or a crushing presence against her body.

A CLOSER LOOK: Widow Makers
Many people believe widows derived their name from their predilection for killing and eating their mates. Those people are correct—but not always: widows very often let their mates go without harming them.

Black Widow Envenomation
Victims almost never feel the bite of the widow's sharp fangs, although a few have reported immediate piercing pain. There may be little or no redness and swelling at the site initially, but a small, red, slightly hard bump may form later. Sometimes the bite site remains elusive,

making a final diagnosis of spider bite difficult. Within thirty to sixty minutes, systemic symptoms may become disturbingly dramatic. Pain and anxiety become intense. Severe muscular cramping and rigidity often center in the large muscles of the abdomen, lower back, and limbs. Facial swelling may occur. Watch for headaches, nausea, vomiting, dizziness, heavy sweating, and weakness—all common reactions. Weakness of the respiratory muscles has led to death.

Even though victims tend to fear they are dying—and then fear they will not die but live on in extreme pain— black widows kill very few humans. In fact, no deaths from a black widow bite have occurred during many years. The dead are almost always the very young, the very old, or the very unhealthy.

What to Do: Widow Spider Bites

Keep the victim as calm as possible—which, come to think of it, is almost always a good thing to do. If you can find the bite site, wash it and apply an antiseptic such as povidone-iodine. Cooling the injury, with ice if possible or with water or wet compresses if necessary, will reduce the pain. Cold also reduces circulation, which slows down the spread of the venom. Medications for pain, if available, would be appropriate. Strong medications for pain are often deeply appreciated by the victim.

Evacuation to a medical facility is strongly advised, especially if you are unsure what is causing the symptoms. People in severe pain are poor wilderness companions anyway. Most people will receive painkillers and muscle relaxants in the hospital, especially during the initial eight to twelve hours when the agony tends to peak, and one to three days of in-hospital observation. Youngsters, oldsters, and the very sick may be hospitalized longer. Complete recovery is expected, although pain may last for a week or more. Antivenin is available if needed.

Brown Spiders

Another potentially serious spider bite in the United States comes from a brown spider (genus *Loxosceles*), the most famous being *Loxosceles reclusa,* the true brown recluse spider. At least three other species are resident in the United States, all members of the family Sicariidae, the recluse family. Some are called fiddlebacks and some violin spiders, and it really does not matter except to spider lovers. They almost all have the shape of a violin on the top front portion of their body. The head of this "fiddle" points toward the rear of the spider. Generally you will see them colored pale brown to reddish with long slender legs about 1 inch (2 to 3 cm long). Unlike the black widow, both sexes of brown spiders are dangerous.

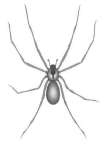

Brown Recluse Spider

Brown spiders prefer the dark and dry places of the South and southern Midwest, but travel comfortably in the freight of trucks and trains, and may possibly be found somewhere in all fifty states. But seeing a brown spider is an uncommon thing, and some experts believe they are not as widespread as once thought. They probably don't bite as often as once thought either. That said, they do not mind living near humans, and they will set up housekeeping underneath furniture, within hanging curtains, and in the shadowed corners of closets. In the wild they hide away during daylight hours beneath rocks, dead logs, and pieces of bark in forests. Solitary and "reclusive" by nature, they roam and hunt at night. They bite more readily in the warmer months, usually at night and only when intentionally or, more often, unintentionally threatened.

Brown Spider Envenomation

Most bitten humans complain of sharp and stinging pain when the brown spider bites—although, as with many spiders, the bite can be painless and the victim unaware. Having relatively dull fangs, the wounds they inflict are often on tender areas of the human anatomy. Initial pain eases off, usually within eight hours, to leave aching and perhaps itching as a replacement. A painful red blister appears where the fangs injected venom. Watch for the development of a bluish circle around the blister and a red, irritated circle beyond that—the characteristic "bull's-eye" lesion of the brown spider. The victim may suffer chills, fever, a generalized weakness, and a diffuse rash.

Sometimes the lesion resolves harmlessly over the next week or two. Sometimes it spreads irregularly as an enzyme in the spider's venom destroys the cells of the victim's skin and subcutaneous fat. Then the ulcerous tissue heals slowly and leaves a lasting scar. In a few children, death may have occurred from severe complications in their circulatory system.

What to Do: Brown Spider Bites

As with many spider bites, the absence of an eight-legged corpse as evidence makes it difficult to be sure exactly what is causing the problem. Initially there is little to be done other than calming the victim and applying cold to the site of the bite for reduction of pain. The presence of systemic responses—such as fever and weakness—should initiate a quick trip to a doctor. Ulcerous skin lesions should also be seen by a physician as soon as possible. Antibiotic therapy usually cures the problem.

Hobo Spiders

The hobo spider (*Tegenaria agrestis*) was accidentally imported from Europe, probably into Seattle and probably in the early 1900s. The species has now spread across the northwestern United States, up into Alaska, and down into Utah. All hobo spiders are light brown, sometimes appearing to have a slightly green/yellow tint, with eight conspicuously hairy legs. The legs range from 1 to 1.5 inches (1.25 to 3.75 cm) in length. A herringbone-stripe pattern in brown, gray, tan, or a mixture of those colors often appears on the abdomen. Hobo spiders have been mistaken for brown spiders (the recluses) and are sometimes called Northwestern brown spiders. Hobos lack the violin shape. Some experts state that the female is more toxic, and some the male, but the dominant belief today is that the male is more toxic in terms of the necrotic (death) response in tissue. It is difficult to tell, and probably irrelevant, which sex you are looking at without special training and really keen eyesight.

Bites from hobo spiders are considered rare by most experts. Hobos tend to avoid large cities and congregate in small towns and rural communities. They like it under houses and deep in woodpiles and clumps of debris. Indoors they may lurk anyplace that is not regularly cleaned. It would be most unusual to find one in distant, untrammeled places. They do not bite unless trapped against the skin of an unsuspecting human with no way to escape.

Hobo Spider Envenomation

Studies of hobo spider venom have been controversial and limited. Tests on rabbits show clear evidence of systemic poisoning from *Tegenaria* venom. It seems as if the bite of a hobo produces a lesion that ulcerates in approximately 50 percent of human victims. It looks like the lesion of a *Loxosceles* bite, and often no one ever knows for sure which kind of spider bit. Visual disturbances, disorientation, or both in victims have been blamed on hobo spider venom, but the most common complaints are headache, muscle weakness, and lethargy.

What to Do: Hobo Spider Bites

No specific treatment has ever been developed for hobo spider bites. Follow the general guidelines for the management of brown spider bites (see page 69).

What to Do: Prevention of Spider Bites

1. Do not try to pick up or capture spiders.
2. Check places you intend to put your hands and feet before exposing your body part to a bite.
3. Gather firewood before dark, or do it carefully while using a flashlight.
4. In dangerous spider country, keep your tent zipped closed.
5. If you must move around in the dark, wear boots or camp shoes.
6. Take a look in your boots before stuffing in your feet in the morning.

A CLOSER LOOK: Tarantulas

Due to a fierce appearance and perhaps even more fierce reputation, entirely undeserved, North American tarantulas (family Theraphosidae) deserve mention and will be given a few words here. The most important words are these: *they are relatively harmless.* Pain, usually mild, seldom more than moderate, typically follows the bite. Later signs and symptoms, such as weakness or collapse of the human victim, are rare, but they are cause for seeking a physician's attention. Fatalities in humans do *not* result from a tarantula bite.

Care for any tarantula wound by washing and dressing it. Cold application, medications for pain, or both would be appropriate treatment.

Several species of tarantulas, including some of those in North America, have unusual and specialized barbed hairs that can be left in human skin. The hairs cause itchy bumps that may be bothersome for weeks. These hairs can be—and should be—removed with any sticky tape. Topical anti-itch medications could be helpful.

Ticks

Unlike spiders, ticks are arachnids that pass diseases to humans. Only mosquitoes, worldwide, transmit diseases more often to humans—and ticks pass a greater variety of diseases.

Ticks are either hard (family Ixodidae) or soft (family Argasidae). If you get sick from a tick in North

America, you probably got bitten by an Ixodid tick. The bites of Argasid ticks rarely cause a problem.

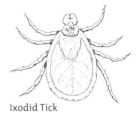

Ixodid Tick

Ixodid ticks molt through three feeding stages: larval (when, by the way, they have only six legs), nymph, and adult. The three stages span a total of about two years. Ixodid ticks can pass disease-causing germs in any stage. They almost always drop off their host between feedings and search out another host later. They will feed on just about anything with blood—mammals, birds, and reptiles.

After finding a host, a tick may search for hours before choosing a spot in which to settle and eat. With specialized pincerlike organs, the tick digs a small, painless wound in the host. Into the wound goes a feeding apparatus called a hypostome, and a relatively powerful sucking mechanism allows the tick to then ingest the blood of the host. Anchored firmly in the wound, an Ixodid tick feeds for an average of two to five

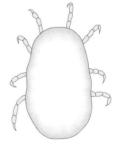

Argasid Tick

days, and sometimes longer than five days, depending on the species. (Argasid ticks, by the way, usually feed to satiation in ten to thirty minutes.) If they pick up germs from one host, they will pass these germs to their next host, but transmission of infection is frequently delayed following tick attachment, sometimes for more than twenty-four hours.

A CLOSER LOOK: The Eating Habits of Ticks
Most ticks consume a single adult blood meal during their lives. A female must be engorged on blood to lay her eggs. She will gain up to fifty times her body weight while engorging.

What to Do: Tick Removal

All ticks should be removed from the host as soon as they are found. While free ranging, ticks can be easily removed, but once attached no simple, effective, approved method of causing the tick to detach itself is known. The best method for removal of an attached tick—and the only method approved by the Centers for Disease Control—is to gently grasp the animal with sharp-tipped tweezers as close as possible to the point of attachment, and remove by applying gentle traction. Grasp the tick perpendicular to its longitudinal axis. Grasping along its axis may turn the tick into a syringe, squirting its germy contents into you. Do not twist the tick. Do not jerk the tick. With slow, gentle traction, it is virtually impossible to tear off the embedded part of the tick—but if it happens the chance of disease transmission from the part left behind is extremely small. A tiny piece of skin may come off painlessly with the tick, which almost always means tick removal is complete. Every effort should be made to avoid crushing the tick and contaminating either victim or helper with crushed tick material. After removal, the wound should be cleansed with soap and water or an antiseptic, and an adhesive strip bandage should be applied. Tweezers should be disinfected after use. If possible, the tick should be preserved for later identification if you get sick.

Tick Poison

Some ticks secrete toxins or venoms that, on one end of the clinical spectrum, cause a relatively mild local reaction ranging from an itchy bump to a rather large red area. Pajaroello ticks (genus *Ornithodoros*), for instance, are greatly feared for their poison in some locales, but the bite is rarely serious. If the wound from any tick bite will not heal, find a doctor.

On the other end of the spectrum, the victim may develop serious complications and even die. Tick paralysis (tick toxicosis) results from venom secreted in the saliva of at least forty-three species of ticks. Occurring most often in the Pacific Northwest and the Rocky Mountains, tick paralysis begins with leg weakness, usually three days or so after the offending tick has attached. An ascending, flaccid paralysis follows, which progressively worsens as long as the tick is attached to the victim (usually a child). Speech dysfunction and difficulty swallowing are late signs, and death from aspiration or respiratory paralysis may occur. Removal of the tick results in a progressive return to normal neurologic function. Both diagnostically and therapeutically, early and meticulous examination for embedded ticks is mandatory.

Tick-Borne Diseases

In the United States at least eight tick-borne illnesses are considered indigenous, including tick paralysis (see above). The diseases include but are not limited to babesiosis, Colorado tick fever, ehrlichiosis, Lyme disease, relapsing fever, Rocky Mountain spotted fever, southern tick-associated rash illness, and tularemia.

Babesiosis

Tick-transmitted protozoan parasites of the genus *Babesia* cause the disease babesiosis, a malaria-like illness. Although the disease is on the rise in America, most cases—but not all—have been limited to the northeastern United States. Typically the patient suffers a slow onset of fatigue, general malaise, and loss of appetite. A few days to a week or so later, fever, sweats, and achy muscles are common. Most people recover without any specific therapy, but unusual fatigue may hang on for much longer than anyone appreciates, and a regimen of drugs may be required for the really sick.

Colorado Tick Fever

This disease is an acute, benign viral infection that occurs throughout the western third of the United States during spring and summer. It is characterized by a sudden onset of fever followed by muscle aches, severe headaches, loss of appetite, nausea, vomiting, and lethargy. There is no specific therapy. The sufferer suffers until the disease runs its course, a time period that can run to several weeks. Once over the illness, the recovered individual probably now has lifelong immunity.

Ehrlichiosis

Two forms of ehrlichiosis may affect humans: human monocytic ehrlichiosis (HME) and human granulocytic ehrlichiosis (HGE). Infected ticks must feed for a minimum of thirty-six hours to pass enough of the bacteria to cause the illnesses. The flu-like condition is characterized, in HME and HGE, by a persistently high fever, headache, muscle aches, gastrointestinal distress, and joint pain. Rashes sometimes occur, more commonly with HME. Most patients recover after a depressing month-long illness and treatment with antibiotics, but some years as many as 70 percent of those affected require hospitalization—in which case the percentage of people who die is almost as high as with Rocky Mountain spotted fever (see below), especially in the elderly or immunocompromised.

Lyme Disease

Lyme disease is an inflammatory illness caused by *Borrelia burgdorferi* bacteria, and it accounts for, according to some experts, approximately 90 percent of tick-borne illnesses in the United States. The number of cases is probably on the rise. Areas of high risk are the Northeast, the upper Midwest, California, southern Oregon, and western Nevada. Most cases develop between early May and the end of November. The first abnormality is far more often than not (occurring in 60 to 80 percent of cases) an expanding, well-defined red rash. The rash migrates: it fades from one area to appear in another. There is no relationship between where the tick bit and where the rash appears. Flu-like symptoms often develop shortly after the rash appears and even if the rash fails to appear. Months after the initial infection, if untreated, arthritis may develop, usually affecting the knees and shoulders. Persistent and varied neurologic abnormalities may occur and persist for years.

It takes more than twenty-four hours of attachment for the tick to pass enough bacteria to cause the disease. Early removal means no illness. Medications shorten the duration of Lyme disease once it is established, and they often prevent later problems.

Relapsing Fever

Relapsing fever is an acute febrile illness caused by *Borrelia* bacteria. Infected ticks, previously attached to wild rodents, are the prime vectors for this disease. Clinically, initial symptoms are those of an acute flu-like illness, but bouts continue at weekly intervals. The diagnosis is established by identification of the organism in blood smears. Antibiotics knock down the germs for good. Prophylactically, one should avoid staying in rodent-infested areas, especially in old abandoned cabins.

Rocky Mountain Spotted Fever

In many areas, but, despite the name, especially in the eastern third of the United States, ticks can transmit unique bacteria of the genus *Rickettsia,* causing Rocky Mountain spotted fever (RMSF), an illness characterized initially by fever, headache, sensitivity to bright light, and muscle aches. On the third to fourth day of fever, a pink rash usually appears and may cover a large percentage of the body. If not treated promptly with antibiotics, the disease may be lethal. RMSF, in fact, currently kills between 3 and 5 percent of those infected. It is indeed the most often fatal tick-borne disease in the United States.

Southern Tick-Associated Rash Illness

Since the middle of the 1980s, rashes similar to the rash of early Lyme disease have appeared on tick-bitten people of the south-central and southeastern United States. At first thought to be Lyme—most signs and symptoms are similar—the disease has recently been tagged with its own name: southern tick-associated rash illness

(STARI). Although research is just getting started, the sick typically get well without intervention. Some physicians, however, suggest a course of oral antibiotics.

Tularemia

Since 1967 fewer than two hundred cases per year of tularemia have been diagnosed in the United States. Though certainly once a disease associated with contact with unhealthy rabbits, ticks are now, by far, considered the prime transmission mode for the bacteria. Although many species of ticks have been incriminated, dog ticks and lone star ticks rank as the most common reservoirs. (Rabbits still qualify as the second most common vector, but you must handle infected tissue, as you might do by skinning and eviscerating a little bunny. Wearing rubber gloves will prevent transmission. You very rarely could also pick up the disease in water or soil by direct contact with, ingestion of, or breathing in contaminated dust or water particles.)

About 80 percent of tularemia cases appear as red bumps that harden and ulcerate, usually on the lower extremities where the tick bit. Ulcers are typically painful and tender. Enlarged, tender lymph nodes are common. The second most common form of tularemia, the typhoidal form, causes fever, chills, and debility. Weight loss may be significant. Pneumonia is a relatively common complication of tularemia. The treatment of choice is antibiotics.

What to Do: Prevention of Tick Bites

1. Do not camp in places where you know ticks are running rampant.

2. Wear light-colored clothing. Wear long-sleeved shirts and long pants tucked inside a pair of high socks. The tick seen early is the tick picked off before it finds your skin.

3. Avoid contact with tall grass and brush whenever possible.

4. Apply a permethrin-based tick repellent (actually an insecticide) to clothing prior to exposure, with particular attention to the ends of shirt sleeves and pants and around the collar area.

5. Apply a repellent containing DEET (a concentration no greater than 30 percent is recommended) to exposed areas of skin.

6. Perform twice-daily (morning and evening), full-body inspection for ticks—and immediately remove all free-ranging and embedded ticks. Note, please, that ticks embed about 20 percent of the time on anatomical spots that the human host cannot easily investigate on his or her own. The message: you need a partner for a total-body tick check.

Scorpions

Although experts disagree on the number of species of scorpions on Earth, they agree that at least thirty species, all in the family Buthidae, carry venom that can kill

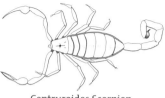

Centruroides Scorpion

a human. From small ones that reach maturity at 0.75 inch to humongous 9-inchers, all scorpions have a somewhat lobsterlike appearance with four pairs of legs and a pair of pincers with which they grab and hold onto their prey. Insects are their primary source of food, but some species will kill and devour small lizards. In all culinary cases, they consume the juices and liquefied tissues of their prey, discarding the solid parts. They inhabit terrain, worldwide, where the temperature stays fairly warm, and are active at night.

FASCINATING FACT
Uniquely, all scorpions "glow" when illuminated by ultraviolet light, such as a black light.

Some scorpions might be able to bite, but that fact is completely insignificant. Significant is the sting they are capable of delivering with the tip of their "tail" by arching it over their backs. A scorpion's tail is actually an extension of the abdomen, and both stinger and venom glands reside in the tail.

Bark Scorpions

In the United States, where about forty scorpion species reside, only *Centruroides exilicauda*—sometimes called the bark scorpion—packs a punch with potential for human death. Found throughout Arizona, bark scorpions are also seen in Texas, New Mexico, and, to a much lesser degree, parts of California and Nevada. No more than around 2 inches (5 cm) in length, they are lean, described sometimes as "streamlined," and have slender pincers. Sometimes colored uniformly tan or brown, they probably appear yellowish most often.

Scorpion Envenomation

Most victims in the United States report no more pain from any scorpion sting than from an irritated honeybee sting. An attack by the genus *Centruroides* may be different. The sting, immediately and exquisitely painful, is increased a lot by a light tap on the site. If the scorpion was *Centruroides,* post-sting manifestations may include tingling in the extremities, heavy sweating, difficulty swallowing, blurred vision, loss of bowel control, and jerky muscular reflexes—indeed, the victim may writhe uncontrollably. Respiratory distress—and death—are possible.

The really bad things that can happen after a *Centruroides* sting typically peak at about five hours after envenomation. With small children, especially infants, the symptoms can be raging in as little as fifteen minutes, and small children, as always, are at much greater risk for a serious reaction. Between the years 1929 and 1954, in Arizona, where *Centruroides* stings are decidedly most common, sixty-nine deaths were reportedly due to bark scorpion stings. Despite the possible complications, in Arizona the last confirmed human death by scorpion was in 1968.

What to Do: Scorpion Envenomations

Even though scorpion envenomations have long been known and dealt with, very little specific treatment has been studied. First aid for any scorpion sting may involve cooling the wound, which may allow the body to more easily break down the molecular structure of the venom. Cooling also reduces pain. Use ice or cool running water if available. On a warm night, a wet compress will help. Keep the victim calm and still. Panic and activity speed up the venom's spread.

Systemic reactions to a *Centruroides* sting are cause for quick evacuation to a medical facility. But even then the standard care provided is supportive: painkillers, fluids, maintenance of normal body temperature, and attention to the other daily needs of the patient. Almost all victims notice marked improvement in nine to thirty hours, although pain and tingling can persist for as long as two weeks. Antivenin is available but usually withheld in the absence of very serious complications, and many experts consider its use controversial at best.

What to Do: Prevention of Scorpion Stings

1. Do not try to pick up or capture scorpions.
2. Check places you intend to put your hands and feet before exposing your body part to a sting.
3. Gather firewood before dark, or do it carefully while using a flashlight.
4. In scorpion country, keep your tent zipped up.
5. If you must move around in the dark, wear boots or camp shoes.
6. Look inside your boots and shake out your clothing before dressing. These are places where scorpions like to hide.

INSECTS

In the class Insecta—animals with six legs and three-part bodies—more than one million species have been named. Probably millions more have not yet been named. Insects make up about one-half of all known organisms, and included in the number are the animals most deadly to humans.

Mosquitoes

Only the female mosquito, which requires a blood feast in order to produce eggs, bites. She will consume up to her body weight with each meal, feeding once every three to four days. If you are the food source, she probably "sees" you first. Closer in she "smells" you—carbon dioxide and lactic acid are being studied as highly likely attractants. Your heat and body moisture are the final, ir-resistible lures. Her bite may sting and later itch, but the really bad news is this: when she sucks out your blood she may leave disease-causing germs behind. (Male mosquitoes, in case you wonder, are vegetarians.)

No creature, great or small, human or nonhuman, has had or continues to have a more significant impact on human beings than mosquitoes. Sure they are bothersome, but consider this: experts estimate that more than 700 million people on Earth will contract a mosquito-borne disease in the next year, and one of every seventeen humans currently alive will die because of a mosquito bite—not the bite, exactly, but the disease caused by the bite. Those diseases include but are not limited to malaria, dengue fever, several forms of encephalitis, yellow fever, and West Nile virus. True, you are not at much risk unless you leave the United States and travel to tropical and subtropical environs. But you are not completely safe near home.

FASCINATING FACTS

1. Mosquitoes bite men more often than they bite women.

2 Mosquitoes bite adults more often than they bite children.

3. Mosquitoes bite overweight people more often than they bite slim people.

West Nile Virus

In Uganda, 1937, the first case of West Nile virus was officially identified. But no known case appeared in the United States until the summer of 1999. Since that first victim in the New York City area, the disease has been diagnosed in humans and, as of 2009, in every state except Alaska, Hawaii, Maine, Vermont, and New Hampshire.

Mosquitoes seem to get the virus from infected birds and maintain it in their salivary glands—then spread it to humans when the insects bite and feed. West Nile virus has also been found in horses, cats, bats, chipmunks, squirrels, skunks, and domestic rabbits, but there is no evidence that humans get the virus from those animals without a mosquito serving as the go-between. There is no evidence that any other arthropod can pass the disease. *Humans cannot pass the disease to other humans.*

Cases of West Nile virus in humans are definitely on the rise, but less than one in five people who contract the disease develop any signs or symptoms. If the signs and symptoms develop, it takes three to fourteen days (five to fifteen days say some experts) after inoculation, and they are almost always mild and flu-like; symptoms may include fever, headache, muscle aches, and, occasionally, a rash on the trunk of the body and swollen lymph glands. These indications of illness most often are harmless and sometimes go away within a few days.

In rare cases, however—approximately one in one hundred fifty—the virus can cross the blood-brain barrier and cause a serious inflammation of the brain (known as West Nile encephalitis); a serious inflammation of the membranes surrounding the brain and the spinal cord (known as West Nile meningitis); or a serious inflammation of the brain and its surrounding membranes (known as West Nile meningoencephalitis). Serious signs and symptoms may include headache, high fever, neck stiffness, stupor, disorientation, coma, tremors, convulsions, muscle weakness, and paralysis. In severe cases problems may persist for weeks, neurological effects may be permanent, and death may result. The chances of death are greater by far if you are over fifty years of age or immunocompromised. So far less than 1 percent of the people in the United States who have been proven to have the disease have died.

FASCINATING FACT
Your chances of being struck by lightning are slightly better than your chances of dying of West Nile virus.

What to Do: Treatment of West Nile Virus
If you have been in an area where West Nile virus could be carried by mosquitoes, and you have been bitten by mosquitoes, and you think you could have the virus, you should see a physician as soon as possible. A blood test can confirm the presence of the disease. Unfortunately no specific treatment exists for West Nile virus, but supportive care leads to a complete recovery in most cases.

And once you get West Nile virus, you probably can never get it again.

>> *IMPORTANT NOTE!*

For updates on West Nile virus and other diseases transmitted by bite or sting, you can call the Centers for Disease Control toll free twenty-four hours a day at 888-232-3228, or go to the agency's web site at www .cdc.gov.

What to Do: Treatment of Mosquito Bites

1. Topical anti-itch products will work to reduce the discomfort. Look for products containing benzocaine for pain relief. Steroid creams have little or no effect.
2. Oral antihistamines, available over the counter, will reduce the itching.
3. Wash and then monitor bites that have been scratched open for signs of infection: increasing redness and swelling, increasing pain, red streaks appearing just beneath the skin.

What to Do: Prevention of Mosquito Bites

1. Wear clothing thick enough or woven tightly enough to prevent penetration of the mosquito's biting apparatus.
2. Wear long sleeves and long pants to reduce the amount of skin accessible to mosquitoes.

3. Wear light-colored clothing: khaki and such. Mosquitoes seem to be partial to dark colors, especially blue.
4. Apply permethrin, a safe insecticide, to clothing.
5. Apply an insect repellent to exposed skin.
6. Sleep under mosquito netting or inside tents with mosquito netting.
7. Avoid exposure during prime mosquito-biting time, usually dawn and dusk.
8. Avoid mosquito-prone areas: near standing water, dense vegetation, areas known to be thick with mosquitoes.

Comparing Repellents

A study reported in the *New England Journal of Medicine* (*NEJM*) in 2002 confirmed that nothing repels better than DEET. Repellents containing 23.8 percent DEET kept bugs away for mean complete-protection time of 301.5 minutes (5 hours). In the *NEJM* report, products containing lemon eucalyptus worked second best, repelling bugs for a mean complete-protection time of 120.1 minutes (2 hours). Third place went to a product containing soybean oil that repelled mosquitoes for a mean complete-protection time of 94.6 minutes (1.6 hours).

FASCINATING FACTS

Neither "ultrasonic" devices nor repelling wristbands have been proven to repel mosquitoes. Tests run with more than a hundred drugs, including vitamin C, vitamin B1 (thiamine), and other vitamins, have failed to reveal that anything was repelled. The FDA has stated that all claims for products to repel insects if taken orally are "either false, misleading, or unsupported by scientific data."

DEET
N,N-diethyl-m-toluamide, now called N,N-diethyl-3-methylbenzamide: we can count ourselves fortunate that we only have to ask for it by the common name of DEET. Available since 1957, DEET has been applied to human skin more than an estimated eight billion times. In all those applications, fewer than fifty cases of serious toxic effects have been documented, and three-fourths of those cases resolved without permanent harm to the victim. Many of the toxic cases involved long-term or heavy use of DEET.

General Use Information for DEET-Based Products
1. Read the label carefully before use.
2. Use a concentration of no more than 30 percent. Higher concentrations provide longer protection but *not* better protection.
3. Apply repellent sparingly. Heavy application and saturation are unnecessary. Repeat applications only as necessary.
4. Do not apply over cuts, wounds, or irritated skin, and keep it out of your eyes and mouth. Discontinue if skin irritation develops.

5. Do not apply to children's hands or allow children to handle the product. Kids will smear the repellent into their eyes and mouths.

6. No specific data relate to the use of DEET on children, but the American Academy of Pediatrics recommends a concentration of no more than 10 percent on children ages two to twelve years. Avoid use on children under two years, say some experts, but others say DEET is okay on children under two years if it is used no more than once a day.

7. After exposure ends, wash skin where DEET was applied—and give little kids a bath.

8. Avoid inhaling the aerosol and spray products that contain DEET.

9. Avoid getting DEET on plastic products. It may cause deterioration of the plastic.

Permethrin

Permethrin, originally extracted from chrysanthemum flowers, is a potent insect neurotoxin currently synthesized for human use as an insect repellent. Not really a repellent, permethrin is an insecticide: an insect killer. Within minutes after contact with permethrin-treated clothing, the insect dies. The substance kills mosquitoes, ticks, fleas, flies, lice, and mites. It bonds strongly to the fibers of clothing and, depending on the concentration and application process, can withstand numerous washings, remaining active, in some cases, for years. Permethrin is colorless and odorless and does no harm to vinyl, plastic, or other fabrics. It can be applied to mosquito netting on tents, to sleeping bags, even to window screens at home. After many tests, the experts agree it apparently does no harm to humans, but it does not work as a repellent or insecticide when applied to skin, so it should *not* be applied to human skin.

Bees, Wasps, and Fire Ants

Bees, wasps (including yellow jackets and hornets), and fire ants—all of the order Hymenoptera—are related largely due, in this context, to their habit of injecting venom when they sting. Most humans find the pain extremely annoying, and that is the end of the story. Every year, however, for an estimated fifty to one hundred people in the United States, the sting causes, usually in less than an hour, the end of their life. Some experts guess the fatality rate runs even higher. Death almost always results from anaphylaxis, a severe allergic reaction: in this case, a reaction to the venom.

All the hymenopterans have the biological wherewithal to manufacture, store, and inject their venom, situated in the most posterior section of their anatomy. When they sting, pain is immediate, redness and swelling soon follow, and itching may not be far behind. The pain may be described as "intense," depending on the species that stung, with hornets often responsible for some of the worst pain.

Bees

Honeybees, nonaggressive by nature, lead the swarm as a source of fatalities in humans. Indeed no more potentially deadly animal is found in North America. As many as 15 percent of all humans may have some sensitivity, often mild, to bee venom, and the honeybee, unlike all other stinging insects, has a barbed stinger that rips out of the insect and stays in human skin, continuing to pump venom for up to twenty minutes. Within a day or so of stinging, the bee dies. Though needless to say, here it is: it is important to remove a bee's stinger as soon as possible. Although it was widely and devoutly believed for many years (and still is by some) that squeezing the embedded bee stinger and attached venom sac would squirt more venom into the sting site, the method of removal does not matter in the least. Speed, here, is your best option. Just get the stinger out, any way you can, as fast as you can.

Bumblebees, also toxic, grow to two to three times the size of honeybees. They are not as social as honeybees, typically nesting in small colonies, usually underground, and are generally noted for being mild mannered and not easily disturbed. They seldom sting, their stinger is barbless, and the physiological reaction in humans to bumblebee stings is the same as the reaction to honeybee stings.

Bee venom itself is not very toxic. It is not designed to kill but simply to repel threats. It usually takes forty to fifty simultaneous stings to cause a systemic reaction that will include one or more of the following: vomiting, diarrhea, headache, fever, muscle spasms, breathing difficulty, maybe even convulsions. It takes, depending on the individual who got stung, somewhere between about 500 and 1400 simultaneous stings to cause death by toxicity.

If confronted by a bee or two, stay calm and back away slowly. Bees do not appear to like rapid movements, especially swatting movements. If attacked by a swarm, run for dense cover, lie face down, and cover your head with your hands. Brightly colored summer clothing seems to attract winged insects, especially bees. Tan, light brown, white, and light green appear to have no special appeal. Insect repellents seldom or never repel bees.

A CLOSER LOOK: Bee Stinger Removal

From *The Lancet*, 348:301–302: "Weal size and thus envenomation increased as the time from stinging to removal of the sting increased, even within seconds. There was no difference in the response to stings which were scraped or pinched off after two seconds … immediate treatment of bee stings should emphasize quick removal without concern regarding the method of removal."

"Killer" Bees

The famed "killer" bees, close relatives of honeybees, were introduced to Brazil from Africa sometime around the 1950s because they were thought to be better honey makers in tropical regions. Being committed to swarming often and great at traveling long distances, they entered the extreme southern United States in October 1990. "Killer" bee venom is no more potent than honeybee venom, and the "killer" types actually inject slightly less venom per sting than honeybees. But "killers" are noted for mass attacks by hundreds of individual bees with little provocation—and they will continue the attack for a very long distance once they become agitated. Some experts estimate that approximately sixty human deaths per year are currently caused by "killer" bees. Interesting to note, the honeybee also is not a native American, having been imported from Europe.

Wasps

Wasp family members, including hornets and yellow jackets, are more likely to sting than bees in many regions, at least partially because some species tend to build their nests on or near human dwellings. Only females have stingers. If they feel threatened or if they feel their nest is threatened, they are more aggressive, generally speaking, than bees. Wasp stingers are barbless, and one wasp can inflict multiple stings. Wasp venom is used not only for defense but also for killing prey—but it takes somewhere around a hundred stings to create a potentially fatal reaction in people. Human death by multiple wasp stings is very rare, but death via anaphylaxis from wasp venom—and it only takes one sting—is not rare.

Unlike bees, wasps are predators and scavengers that are attracted to meat and decaying matter. Garbage, in other words, invites them to visit. Their dirty stingers have a higher rate of infection than bee stings, and the site of their stings should be thoroughly cleaned.

Yellow jackets grow to about a centimeter or so (0.6 inch) in length with bright yellow and black stripes. They tend to be bold, persistent, and aggressive, more aggressive than other hymenopterans. A nest may house up to three thousand individuals, and many will swarm out to deliver multiple stings in a brief amount of time if the nest is disturbed.

FASCINATING FACT
The social wasps (such as paper wasps, bald-faced hornets, and yellow jackets) build their nests out of paper. They make the paper by chewing up fragments of wood and leaves that they mix with saliva to construct the elaborate nests.

What to Do: Hymenopteran Stings
The pain of a sting by a hymenopteran is diminished by immediately applying cold to the site. Some topical analgesics also will ease the pain. Antihistamines will reduce the local reaction, both its duration and its extent. Steroid creams may decrease the local reaction,

but no topical medications have proven truly effective for reducing the reaction.

Mild to moderate allergic reactions characterized by hives, facial swelling, and dizziness can be treated with an oral antihistamine. If severe breathing difficulty results, only injectable epinephrine—available by prescription in preloaded syringes—reverses the reaction.

Fire Ants

Ants are found worldwide, and many species are capable of delivering a painful sting. In the United States only one species (*Solenopsis invicta*) carries medical significance in its venom. Way down south, from North Carolina to Florida and across to Texas, in the warm summer months beware of a small reddish-brown to black ant that lives in mounds. Not an indigenous insect, the notoriously aggressive fire ant has spread like kudzu since it first appeared in Alabama in the 1920s. It's not the least bit unusual for a mound to house twenty-five thousand fire ants, and unsuspecting humans who step on a mound can find their legs covered in hundreds of ants within thirty seconds. Unlike most ants, fire ants attack instead of running away.

The ant attaches its sharp mandibles to skin, but the mild pain of the bite only marks the beginning of an enraged fire ant attack. While holding on, the ants jab in their rear-end-positioned stinger and release venom, pull it out, twist, and jab again. They will keep jabbing until you swat. If you do not swat, they will sting a ring of extraordinarily painful burning wounds. Pain usually keeps your teeth clenched for about an hour. Over the next few hours, swelling develops and a clear fluid-filled bump appears. Bumps can itch and hurt for a week.

Although most people get over fire ant stings by cursing and scratching, serious reactions are not uncommon. Deaths due to anaphylaxis from fire ant bites may run as high as thirty humans per year. During the famous Fire Ant Summer of 1971, victims numbering more than six thousand were treated for infections from stings. On the more serious end of treatment that year, seventy-six people had severe allergic responses, eight needed skin grafts, and five had body parts amputated.

What to Do: Fire Ant Bites

If attacked by a hoard of fire ants, running and swatting are both approved methods of fighting back. The application of cold may ease the pain for a short while. Some products claim to ease the symptoms—and you could find they work for you. But a few experts suggest that no medications have proven effective in either relieving the symptoms or preventing the fluid-filled bumps.

What to Do: Anaphylaxis

Anaphylaxis is a true, life-threatening emergency. Breathing difficulty (from airway constriction) or anaphylactic shock (from rapidly dilating blood vessels) that results in a true anaphylactic reaction requires rapid field treatment—or else the victim will die. The ability to reverse fatal anaphylaxis requires administration of epinephrine.

Inhaled epinephrine, a nonprescription drug, may relax the airway enough to be life saving. Unfortunately, inhaled epinephrine will not work if the victim cannot inhale—plus it does little or nothing for shock.

The most specific and valuable treatment is the use of injectable epinephrine that works to alleviate both breathing difficulties and shock. This prescription product is available in kit form. Sometimes one injection is not enough, and rebound or recurrent reactions can occur up to twenty-four hours after the original incident. A second injection should be given in five minutes if the condition of the victim worsens and in fifteen minutes if the condition of the victim does not improve.

Some physicians recommend that three total doses be carried at all times by people who know they are severely allergic, and some physicians recommend carrying four or even more.

Once the victim can breathe and swallow, an oral antihistamine should be given—as soon as the patient can accept the tablets and swallow. Many over-the-counter antihistamines are available, with diphenhydramine currently being most often rec-ommended post-epinephrine. The usual recommended dose of diphenhydramine is 50 to 100 mg to start, and approximately 50 mg every four to six hours until the victim is turned over to definitive medical care. (Check with your physician for optimal doses if you know you are allergic.)

Fleas

Fleas (family Pulicidae) are wingless insects comprised mostly of legs and mouth. They can jump really high and bite really well. Many species live on birds and mammals worldwide, with some feeding on a particular host, some feeding indiscriminately on any host, all feeding on blood. Both sexes are blood feeders and, unlike many arthropods, both will bite several times while feeding instead of the customary hit-and-run tactics of most biters. Fleas are important considerations partly because the bites are uncomfortable and mostly because they can pass diseases to humans, including several forms of plague. In recent years plague has been on the rise in the western United States.

A CLOSER LOOK: The Plague

Between 1347 and 1350, the Black Death, caused by the bacteria *Yersinia pestis,* began somewhere in Asia and eventually rubbed out about twenty-five million Europeans (roughly one-third the population). Nine-tenths of the people of England were permanently laid low. Before those devastating years, even in ancient times, reports of the scourges of plague were known and feared.

Carried by rodents and passed primarily by the bite of rodent fleas, the bacteria that cause plague kill both rodent and flea, an unusual aspect of this disease. Black rats are especially susceptible, and *Rattus rattus* is blamed for the Black Death of the fourteenth century. In the United States, deer mice and various voles harbor the bacteria. The pathogen's presence is amplified in prairie dogs and ground squirrels. Other possible reservoirs include chipmunks, marmots, wood rats, rabbits, and hares. Coyotes and bobcats are known to have transmitted plague to humans while the humans were skinning the dead animals. Skunks, raccoons, and badgers are also suspect during the skinning process.

Meat-eating pets that eat infected rodents (or get bitten by infected fleas) can acquire plague. Dogs do not get very sick, but cats do. There is only one known case of plague being passed from a dog to a human, but several cats have passed the disease to humans by biting them, coughing on them, or carrying their fleas to them. In addition, sick people transmit plague readily to other people.

Types of Plague

Several forms of plague exist, but the three most common are bubonic, septicemic, and pneumonic. Buboes are inflamed, enlarged lymph nodes, and they give bubonic plague its name. After an incubation period of two to six days, patients usually suffer fever, chills, malaise, muscle aches, and headaches. Blackened, bleeding skin sores arise, and they gave a name to the Black Death. The septicemic form may appear similar but does not give rise to buboes—though gastrointestinal pain with nausea, vomiting, and diarrhea is common. The pneumonic form results most often from inhaling droplets that contain the bacteria, but it can develop from bacteria that get into the blood. Coughing with the pneumonic form often produces blood in the sputum of the victim.

What to Do: Treatment and Prevention of Plague

Since fleas will not leave a host until they have fed well, and since you will not be near enough to many wild animals, the chance of getting bitten by a plague-ridden flea is small. Most of the cases reported in recent years have been acquired by people who handled dead animals. Hikers and campers may be at mild risk if they hang around rodent-infested areas.

Flea bites tend to itch a lot, so much that scratching removes the bumps and you may not be sure later that something bit you. If you think you have been bitten by a flea and, within a week, develop a high fever, chills, headache, and muscle aches, you might have the plague—most commonly bubonic plague, similar to the Black Death that ravaged Europe long ago but not as devastating.

If plague is suspected, it should be treated soon by a physician. Fatalities are common today, especially in the pneumonic and septicemic forms. The treatment drug of choice is often streptomycin, injected four times a day for five days.

Prevention includes avoidance of rodents and rodent-rich areas, avoiding touching sick or dead animals (but if you must touch them wear rubber gloves), restraining dogs and cats while traveling in infected areas (because they can pick up infected fleas), and using effective insect repellents.

Say No to Bugs

1. Set camp well away from wet areas and moving or standing water during bug season. Select open areas with little vegetation.
2. Set camp to take advantage of breezes that push away many bugs.
3. Clean up thoroughly after meals, closing and storing anything that might attract bugs.
4. Do not sleep with anything that might attract bugs or other animals: food, garbage, toothpaste, deodorant, soap, or other scented products.
5. Choose unscented camp products: soap, lotion, toilet paper, and so on.
6. Keep your tent door zipped shut.
7. Never approach or try to feed a live animal.
8. Never touch a dead animal.

9. Leave your pets at home—or, if you must take them along, keep them close and under control, and be forewarned that they will bring bugs back to you.

10. Avoid lights at night as much as possible. Many bugs are attracted to light.

11. Before traveling in an area, gather specific information from local land managers and health officials about what diseases might exist there and how to avoid them.

SELECTED REFERENCES

CHAPTER 1: INGESTED POISONS

Graeme, Kimberlie A. "Toxic Plant Ingestions." *Wilderness Medicine*, 5th ed. Philadelphia: Mosby, 2007.

Schneider, Sandra M., and Mark W. Donnelly. "Toxic Mushroom Ingestions." *Wilderness Medicine,* 5th ed. Philadelphia: Mosby, 2007.

Tilton, Buck. *Wilderness First Responder,* 3rd ed. Guilford, CT: The Globe Pequot Press, 2010.

CHAPTER 2: INHALED POISONS

American Association of Poison Control Centers. www.aapcc.org.

Weaver, L. K., et al. "Hyperbaric Oxygen for Acute Carbon Monoxide Poisoning." *New England Journal of Medicine*, 347, no. 14 (Oct. 3, 2002): 1057–1067. www.nejm.org.

CHAPTER 3: ABSORBED POISONS

Anderson, Bryan E., and James G. Marks. "Plant-Induced Dermatitis." *Wilderness Medicine,* 5th ed. Philadelphia: Mosby, 2007.

Wilkerson, James A. *Medicine for Mountaineering & Other Wilderness Activities,* 6th ed. Seattle: The Mountaineers Books, 2010.

CHAPTER 4: INJECTED POISONS

Centers for Disease Control and Prevention (CDC). www .cdc.gov.

Erickson, Timothy B. "Arthropod Envenomation and Parasitism." *Wilderness Medicine,* 5th ed. Philadelphia: Mosby, 2007.

Fradin, Mark, and John Day. "Comparative Efficacy of Insect Repellents Against Mosquito Bites." *New England Journal of Medicine,* 347, no. 1 (July 4, 2002): 13–18. www .nejm.org.

Gold, Barry, et al. "Bites of Venomous Snakes." *New England Journal of Medicine,* 347, no. 5 (August 1, 2002). www.nejm.org.

Norris, Robert, and Sean Bush. "Bites by Venomous Reptiles in the Americas." *Wilderness Medicine,* 5th ed. Philadelphia: Mosby, 2007.

Suchard, Jeffery R. "Scorpion Envenomation." *Wilderness Medicine,* 5th ed. Philadelphia: Mosby, 2007.

ABOUT THE AUTHOR

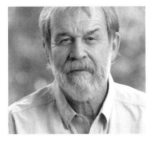

Buck Tilton, MS, WEMT, has more than thirty years of experience in outdoor health and safety. He has taught worldwide, spending most of his adult life instructing outdoor enthusiasts in wilderness medicine. He is co-founder of the Wilderness Medicine Institute of the National Outdoor Leadership School in Lander, Wyoming, and has authored more than 1100 magazine articles and authored or co-authored numerous books including several in the *Don't* series, *Tent & Car Camper's Handbook*, and *Trekker's Handbook*. He lives happily in Lander with his wife Kat, his son Zachary, and his daughter BaoXin Cheyenne.

THE MOUNTAINEERS, founded in 1906, is a nonprofit outdoor activity and conservation club, whose mission is "to explore, study, preserve, and enjoy the natural beauty of the outdoors . . . ." The club sponsors many classes and year-round outdoor activities in the Pacific Northwest and supports environmental causes through educational programs and activities and by sponsoring legislation. The Mountaineers Books supports the club's mission by publishing travel and natural history guides, instructional texts, and works on conservation and history.

Visit www.mountaineersbooks.org to view our complete list of more than 500 outdoor titles.

The Mountaineers Books
1001 SW Klickitat Way, Suite 201
Seattle, WA 98134
800-553-4453
mbooks@mountaineersbooks.org

Leave No Trace strives to educate visitors about the nature of their recreational impacts and offers techniques to prevent and minimize such impacts. Leave No Trace is best understood as an educational and ethical program, not as a set of rules and regulations.

OTHER TITLES YOU MIGHT ENJOY FROM
THE MOUNTAINEERS BOOKS

Don't Die Out There Deck
A compact, full deck of playing cards, with
critical outdoor survival tips on each card

**Backcountry Cooking Deck:
50 Recipes for Camp & Trail**
Dorcas Miller
Delicious trail-ready recipes in
a portable format (4x5½)

**Don't Get Sick: The Hidden
Dangers of Camping and Hiking**
Buck Tilton & Rick Bennett
"[This] book will take up almost no space,
but just might help you avoid big
trouble, even death."—*Dayton News*

**Don't Forget the Duct Tape:
Tips & Tricks for Repairing &
Maintaining Outdoor & Travel Gear,
2nd Edition** *Kristin Hostetter*
"… a must-have for anyone whose outdoor
gear gets loved to death on a regular basis."
—*The Flint Journal*

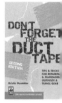

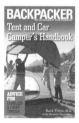

**Tent and Car Camper's Handbook:
Advice for Families & First-Timers**
Buck Tilton, with Kristin Hostetter
"From the absolute basics to the details that can
make a good experience great, these authors
know their stuff and are eager to share it. Their
love and respect for nature is both evident and
contagious, and this book is a pleasure to read."
—*Newsday*

**The Mountaineers Books has more than
500 outdoor recreation titles in print.**
For details, visit
www.mountaineersbooks.org.